Empowerment, Lifelong Learning and Recovery
in Mental Health

Also by Peter Ryan

COMMUNITY SUPPORT FOR MENTAL HEALTH

OCCUPATIONAL STRESS AND THE MANAGEMENT OF VIOLENCE

ASSERTIVE OUTREACH: A STRENGTHS APPROACH TO POLICY AND
PRACTICE

Also by Shulamit Ramon

A STAKEHOLDER'S APPROACH TO INNOVATION IN MENTAL HEALTH
SERVICES: A READER FOR THE 21ST CENTURY (*editor*)

USERS RESEARCHING HEALTH AND SOCIAL CARE: AN EMPOWERING
AGENDA? (*editor*)

MENTAL HEALTH AT THE CROSSROADS: THE PROMISE OF THE
PSYCHOSOCIAL APPROACH (*editor*)

SOCIAL WORK IN THE CONTEXT OF POLITICAL CONFLICT, INTERNATIONAL
ASSOCIATION OF SCHOOLS OF SOCIAL WORK

CUTTING EDGE ISSUES IN COMPARATIVE SOCIAL WORK AND SOCIAL
POLICY RESEARCH (*co-editor*)

Also by Tim Greacen

FOLIE ET JUSTICE (*co-editor*)

SANTE MENTALE DU JEUNE ENFANT: PREVENIR ET INTERVENIR
(*co-editor*)

SAVOIR PARLER AVEC SON MEDECIN: LE GUIDE DE LA NOUVELLE
RELATION PATIENT-MEDECIN

POUR DES USAGERS DE LA PSYCHIATRIE ACTEURS DE LEUR PROPRE VIE:
RETABLISSEMENT, INCLUSION SOCIALE, EMPOWERMENT
(*co-editor*) (forthcoming)

SEXUALITE ET SIDA EN MILIEU SPECIALISE (*co-author*)

Empowerment, Lifelong Learning and Recovery in Mental Health

Towards a New Paradigm

Edited by

Peter Ryan
Middlesex University, UK

Shulamit Ramon
University of Hertfordshire, UK

and

Tim Greacen
Etablissement public de santé Maison Blanche, Paris, France

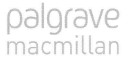

First published 2012 by
PALGRAVE MACMILLAN

Palgrave Macmillan in the UK is an imprint of Macmillan Publishers Limited,
registered in England, company number 785998, of Houndmills, Basingstoke,
Hampshire RG21 6XS.

Palgrave Macmillan in the US is a division of St Martin's Press LLC,
175 Fifth Avenue, New York, NY 10010.

Palgrave Macmillan is the global academic imprint of the above companies
and has companies and representatives throughout the world.

Palgrave® and Macmillan® are registered trademarks in the United States,
the United Kingdom, Europe and other countries.

ISBN 978–0–230–29285–7

This book is printed on paper suitable for recycling and made from fully
managed and sustained forest sources. Logging, pulping and manufacturing
processes are expected to conform to the environmental regulations of the
country of origin.

A catalogue record for this book is available from the British Library.

A catalog record for this book is available from the Library of Congress.

10   9   8   7   6   5   4   3   2   1
21 20 19 18 17 16 15 14 13 12

Printed and bound in Great Britain by
CPI Antony Rowe, Chippenham and Eastbourne

Contents

List of Tables and Figures   vii

Acknowledgements   viii

Notes on Contributors   x

Introduction   1
Peter Ryan, Shulamit Ramon and Tim Greacen

Part I   Recovery

1   Recovery, Lifelong Learning, Empowerment and Social
    Inclusion: Is a New Paradigm Emerging?   15
    Helen Glover

2   TREE: Towards Recovery, Empowerment and Experiential
    Expertise of Users of Psychiatric Services   36
    Wilma Boevink

3   Wellness Recovery Action Planning (WRAP)   50
    Barbara Evans and Kate Sault

4   The Role of Mental Health Service Users in Recovery
    from Professional Stigma   59
    Robert W. Surber

5   Developing Successful Recovery-Oriented Mental
    Health Services   69
    Jed Boardman and Geoff Shepherd

Part II   Social Inclusion and Employment

6   Designing Policies to Foster the Community Inclusion
    of People in Recovery   85
    Larry Davidson, Elizabeth Flanagan and Thomas Styron

7   Employment and Social Inclusion: Implementing the
    Model and Facing the Reality   99
    Justine Schneider

8   Overcoming Barriers to Empowerment   112
    Tim Greacen and Emmanuelle Jouet

Part III   Empowerment and Lifelong Learning

 9 Empowerment: Key Concepts and Evidence Base   135
    Peter Ryan, Anja Esther Baumann and Chris Griffiths

10 Evaluating Service-User Involvement in Mental
    Health Services   146
    David Crepaz-Keay

11 Lifelong Learning, Mental Health and Higher Education:
    a UK Focus   154
    Jill Anderson and Janet Holmshaw

12 Lifelong Learning and Well-Being: The Health Benefits
    of Lifelong Learning for People with Mental Illness   173
    James Ogunleye, Chris Griffiths, Ian Dawson and Klavs Nybjerg

13 Stakeholders' Lifelong Learning and Organisational Change
    Experiences in the Context of the EMILIA Project   189
    Marja Kaunonen and Shulamit Ramon

14 Getting on with Your Life: a User's Experience of
    Participating in the EMILIA Project   204
    Torill Klevan Nilsen

15 Service Users' Experiences of Lifelong Learning   209
    *Irja Nieminen, Torill Klevan Nilsen, Isard Vila,
    María Trinidad Solá and the Fenix Users Group*

16 Mental Health Service Users as Trainers in the Context
    of the EMILIA Project   217
    Terese Stenfors-Hayes and Peter Ryan

Index   232

List of Tables and Figures

Tables

1.1 Historical beliefs influencing current practice   19

1.2 Potential negative impacts of treatment and social environments for people who experience mental illness   23

1.3 Testing service environments' enabling ability: the Star of Recovery Test Questions   32

8.1 Organisations participating in the EMILIA Project at the eight European sites   117

8.2 Seven consecutive surveys on obstacles and facilitators encountered before and during implementation   119

8.3 Examples of Pathways Readiness Evaluation Tool (PRET) checklist items   126

8.4 Examples from the Services and Institutions Readiness Checklist (SIRC)   127

10.1 Service-user involvement indicators   151

Figures

1.1 Star of Recovery   26

16.1 Learning and teaching model   219

Acknowledgements

We would like to acknowledge the influence and inspiration of all the EMILIA teams, both users and staff from the 15 partner sites across Europe, and in particular:

- All service users who participated in the EMILIA project
- Peter Jones, Kate Holmes, Jacquie Lynskey, Paulette Case Robinson, Peter Johnson and Peter Sartori of the service user advisory group at Middlesex University
- Janet Holmshaw and Nicky Torrance at Middlesex University, UK
- Ian Dawson and the Nordland Psychiatric Hospital team in Bodø for their constant and ongoing support throughout the project
- Marja Kaunonen, School of Health Sciences, University of Tampere, Finland
- Emmanuelle Jouet at Hôpital Maison Blanche, Paris; Dominique Granger for her work in formatting the book drafts; and Olivier Las Vergnas, from la Cité des Métiers, Paris.
- Kerstin Bäck Moller, Bettina Hansen and Francisca Sanchez Pedersen from the Department of Education, Psychiatric Services of the County of Aarhus, Denmark
- Czeslaw Czabala, Marta Anczewska and Piotr Switaj from the Institute of Psychiatry and Neurology, Warsaw, Poland
- Marie-Louise Bonnelykke Roberston from the Social and Psychiatry Department of Storstrom County, Denmark
- Arunas Germanavicius and Saulius Peciulis (†) of the Vilnius University Psychiatric Clinic, Lithuania
- Mojca Urek and Vito Flaker from the University of Ljubljana, Slovenia
- Bojan Sosic from HealthNet International, Sarajevo, Bosnia and Herzegovina
- Uno Fors and Terese Stenfors-Hayes from the Karolinska Institute, Stockholm, Sweden
- Stelios Stylianidis, Costandi Lambaki and Panagiotis Chondros from EPAPSY, Scientific Association for Regional Development and Mental Heath, Athens, Greece

- Paz Flores, Roser Izquierdo Aymerich and Eithne Ní Laocha, from the Municipal Institute of Medical Research Foundation, Barcelona, Spain; and
- Stelios Stylianidis, Costandi Lambaki, Panagiotis Chondros and Stella Pantelidou from EPAPSY, Scientific Association for Regional Development and Mental Heath, Athens, Greece

†We acknowledge in particular the contribution which Saulius Peciulis made to the success of the EMILIA Project, who is sadly died the course of the project.

Finally, we would like to acknowledge the contribution of EU framework 6 funding to resource the work of the EMILIA project from 2005–10.

Notes on Contributors

Jill Anderson is senior lecturer in Social Work at the University of Cumbria, UK, and is Senior Project Development Officer for the Mental Health in Higher Education project, which aims to increase networking and the sharing of approaches to learning and teaching about mental health – across the disciplines in higher education. Jill has a background as a mental health social worker and a strong interest in the involvement of service users and carers in the education of health and social care professionals.

Anja Esther Baumann is technical officer for Mental Health at the WHO Regional Office for Europe. Dr. Baumann is responsible for mental health promotion and disorder prevention. Being a long-term advocate for people with mental health problems and their families, she engages particularly in the empowerment of mental health service users and their carers and the fight against stigma and discrimination related to mental illness. Prior to her engagement at the WHO Regional Office for Europe, she worked for ten years in the Psychiatric Clinic/ Department of Psychiatry at the University of Düsseldorf, Germany, on social-psychological aspects of mental illness.

Wilma Boevink is a social scientist and an active member of the Dutch user movement in psychiatry. Until recently she was also a board member of the European Network of (ex-) Users and Survivors of Psychiatry (ENUSP). A long-term user herself, she is one of the founders of TREE, a national user-run enterprise working in the area of recovery, empowerment and experiential expertise of users in mental health services. She is Professor of Recovery at Hanze University, Groningen, the Netherlands, and currently works in the research department at Trimbos Institute, a centre of expertise on mental health and addiction in the city of Utrecht. In 2006, she received the Douglas Bennett Award for her oeuvre. In 2010, the Netherlands Organisation for Health Research and Development designated TREE as 'Pearl project'.

Jed Boardman is specialised in programmes for the social inclusion of people with disabilities and benefits allocated to them. He is also Chair of the General and Community Faculty of the Royal College of Psychiatrists in London, UK.

David Crepaz-Keay is current Head of Empowerment and Social Inclusion at the Mental Health Foundation, London, UK. As a service user with over 20 years' experience in service user involvement, he has occupied a number of prestigious posts including chief executive of Mental Health Media, vice-chair for the Commission for Patient and Public Involvement in Health, founding member of National Survivor User Network and former chair and treasurer of Survivors Speak Out. He is also advisor to World Health Organisation Europe on empowerment.

Larry Davidson is Professor of Psychology at the University of Yale, Department of Psychiatry, USA, where he directs the Recovery and Community Health programme. His research deals with the psychosocial rehabilitation of people living with mental health disorders and the recovery process, in particular for people with psychosis.

Ian Dawson is trained as both a psychiatric nurse and social worker, and is currently the co-ordinator of services at Salten Psychiatric Centre, Bodø in Northern Norway. Ian has worked mainly in adult psychiatry in the last 30 years, both in England and Norway. He is the researcher and work package leader for dissemination in the EMILIA project.

Barbara Evans trained as a social worker and currently works for Hampshire County Council as a Workforce Development Advisor for Mental Health. She works to ensure service user and carer voices are heard within the learning context and was instrumental in commissioning a 100 per cent service-user training organisation in Hampshire, UK.

The Fenix Users Group are members of the "Association 'Fenix' for mutual help in mental distress", a user organization established in 2000 in the city of Tuzla in Bosnia and Herzegovina. The members of Fenix played a key role in Bosnia throughout the EMILIA project. Today, Fenix, which is involved in a number of projects both nationally and abroad, is run by users alone, with no input from professionals, other than as employees.

Elizabeth Flanagan is an assistant professor in the Department of Psychiatry, Yale School of Medicine, USA. She is a faculty member for the Yale Program for Recovery and Community Health. Dr. Flanagan's personal research programme investigates stigma and discrimination towards people with mental illness, especially in mental health and primary care settings. She also researches the first-person experience of mental illness and seeks to revise the Diagnostic and Statistical Manual of Mental Disorders (DSM) and the International Classification of Diseases (ICD) so that they accurately represent the personal experience of mental illness.

Helen Glover is a social worker, originally from Australia. She uses her professional skills and experience as a user to promote the establishment of mental health services focused on the concept of recovery. In 2001, she participated in drafting relevant sections on this topic in the Report from the National Institute of Mental Health of England (NIMHE).

Tim Greacen is a psychologist and director of the Maison Blanche Research Laboratory, Paris, France. In addition to the EMILIA Project, he is currently managing projects on access to mental healthcare for excluded social groups, mental health promotion in children and adults and users' participation in mental healthcare. He teaches regularly at the Universities of Paris and Montpellier and the Ecole Centrale in Paris.

Chris Griffiths has worked on two Europe-wide European Union-funded mental health projects, as a researcher in Improving Access to Psychological Therapies (IAPT) service, and as a lecturer at university undergraduate level. His work has focused on the empowerment, social inclusion, employment, lifelong learning and mental health promotion for mental health service users.

Janet Holmshaw is a Senior Lecturer in Mental Health at Middlesex University, UK, where she teaches social inclusion and recovery in mental health, mental health law and ethics. She is the project leader for service user and carer involvement in teaching and learning on the mental health programmes. Janet's background is in nursing and research (both mainly in mental health) and teaching medical sociology, medical law and ethics and mental health.

Emmanuelle Jouet is a specialist in educational sciences. She works in the field of training programmes for mental health service users and is currently researcher for the EMILIA project at the Maison Blanche Research Laboratory in Paris, France.

Marja Kaunonen is adjunct professor, School of Health Sciences at the University of Tampere, Finland and is the EMILIA Project research leader since March 2008. Her research interests include grief and bereavement, support of families and individuals in challenging life situations and nursing administration and management.

Irja Nieminen is a doctoral candidate at the School of Health Sciences, University of Tampere, Finland. She previously worked as a researcher in the EMILIA project. Her doctoral research focuses on mental health service users' participation in training: one of the training programmes developed in the EMILIA project is tested in Finland.

Torill Klevan Nilsen is a member of Mental Health, a user organisation in Norway and has personal user experience. She was a key user representative in the EMILIA project and has been leading EMILIA training in Bodø.

Klavs Nybjerg is an occupational health psychologist and senior educational consultant at Aarhus University Hospital. He has been a researcher for the EMILIA project in Aarhus, Denmark.

James Ogunleye led the UK contribution to the EMILIA project's Lifelong Learning Workpackage. He is a recognised expert in the field of lifelong learning education. Currently, he serves on the European Commission's Panel of Experts – project scrutineer/reviewer – on the Lifelong Learning Programme 2007–13. He chairs the Lifelong Learning, Higher Education and Social Inclusion thematic section of two annual international conferences based respectively in Eastern Europe and the Mediterranean.

Shulamit Ramon is Professor of Mental Health Research at the University of Hertfordshire, UK. With a background of researching mental health in Europe, she is currently managing two research projects, on shared decision making in psychiatric medication management, and on domestic violence and mental health in Europe. She has published 11 books, most recently *Cutting Edge Issues in Comparative Social Work and Social Policy* (2009).

Peter Ryan is Professor of Mental Health at Middlesex University, UK, and chair of ENTER Mental Health, a European mental health network. He is a social worker by background. He was chief investigator for the EMILIA Project (2005–10) and currently co-ordinates PROMISE, a European mental health promotion project. He has published four books, over 80 articles and has specialist research interests in lifelong learning in mental health, mental health promotion and occupational mental health.

Kate Sault is WRAP co-ordinator, a role she developed within the Southern Health Trust, UK. She originally trained as a Mental Health Nurse and worked in an inpatient unit for several years before becoming WRAP co-ordinator and has spent the past six years working with others to develop more recovery-orientated services including training staff and service users in recovery and WRAP.

Justine Schneider is a social researcher and social worker. She is currently Professor of Mental Health and Social Care at the Institute of Mental Health, University of Nottingham, UK. She has a long-standing research interest in employment for people with disabilities, and also conducts research in many aspects of applied health and social care, including psychosocial interventions, carer strain, dementia services and stigma.

Geoff Shepherd is a policy advisor to the employment programme team at Sainsbury Centre for Mental Health (SCMH), UK. He has a particular interest in commissioning issues and in measuring work and employment outcomes. He also has experience of developing a user employment programme ('leading by example' in a mental health trust and in promoting joint training between staff in mental health services and those in jobcentre plus offices. Mr. Shepherd is currently involved in the project run by an independent sector provider (Richmond Fellowship Employment and Training) to evaluate the impact of 'employment specialists' in primary care.

María Trinidad Solá and ISARD VILA are users and co-trainers in the EMILIA programme in Barcelona, Catalonia, Spain.

Terese Stenfors-Hayes is a specialist in the field of medical education. She previously worked as an educational developer at Karolinska Institutet, Sweden. She led the work on lifelong learning in the EMILIA project and is currently employed as a researcher at the University of British Columbia, Canada.

Thomas Styron is a clinical psychologist and Associate Professor of Psychiatry at the Yale School of Medicine, USA. Dr. Styron serves as executive director of the Community Services Network of Greater New Haven, a collaborative of 18 community-based not-for-profit organisations which provide a broad array of integrated community supports, include housing, employment and social opportunities, for individuals with serious mental illness. Dr. Styron's research and teaching focuses on best practices in the area of recovery-oriented care for individuals with serious mental illnesses. Dr. Styron is based at the Connecticut Mental Health Center, a public psychiatric hospital under the auspices of Yale's Department of Psychiatry, where he directs the psychology training programme for the hospital's outpatient services division.

Robert W. Surber is a clinical professor with the University of California San Francisco, Department of Psychiatry, and principal of Robert Surber Consultation in Behavioral Health, located in San Francisco, California, and Keaau, Hawaii, USA. His expertise is in implementing the evidence-based practices that have been demonstrated to promote recovery with a focus on the role of consumers in delivering mental health and substance abuse treatment services. He has provided consultation and training in these areas to 145 organisations throughout the United States as well as in Europe and Asia.

Introduction

Peter Ryan, Shulamit Ramon and Tim Greacen

The chapters that follow offer a European and international perspective on empowerment, lifelong learning, social inclusion and recovery in mental health. In particular, they explore the contribution that lifelong learning – a hitherto neglected concept in the area of mental health – can make in linking these concepts into a coherent whole. The thesis of the book is that these four concepts are closely connected. We believe that together they contribute to a new paradigm in mental health, one that locates the service user as the central driver of their own life, a life of their own choosing, in a community in which they are citizens with equal rights to all other citizens and with mental health services configured so as to support this process rather than perpetuating the traditional 'client' or 'patient' roles.

The field of mental health is undergoing a considerable paradigm shift in terms of rethinking core issues that, until recently, have been taken for granted, such as chronicity, deficits and strengths, capability for social inclusion, peer support, education, training and employment, and the meaning of empowerment and recovery from mental illness. Inevitably, a change of this magnitude within a complex system in which mental health services operate everywhere attracts responses ranging from the enthusiastic right through to the dismissive and hostile. How to enable service providers, users, carers and the general public to be open to the possibilities this shift can lead to, and to actively participate in the process of this change, forms a central part of the contributions to this book.

Despite promising beginnings, the evidence-based knowledge of how to achieve empowerment, recovery, social inclusion and the potential contribution of lifelong learning is at its infancy. As these notions become increasingly recognised across Europe, and indeed internationally, more and more service users are participating as partners in many aspects of health and social care delivery, policymaking and professional training. While there are recent publications on recovery (Slade 2009, Repper and Perkins 2003), relatively less has been produced on empowerment (Barnes and Bowl 2000) and less still on lifelong learning in terms of its links and application to mental health.

This book explores new ground in identifying the barriers and obstacles to empowerment as well as good practice examples in developing effective approaches to integrating these concepts in both mental health services and educational institutions. In particular, the book highlights the role lifelong learning can play in offering a bridge to the achievement of recovery. The mutual benefits of this approach to all stakeholders are emphasised, without glossing over the difficulties inherent in it, and it will, we hope, be relevant and of interest to a wide audience including health and social service professionals and managers, service users and those involved in higher education.

The book is divided into three interlinked sections. The first gives an overview of recovery. The second focuses on the closely linked issues of social inclusion and employment. The third part views empowerment and lifelong learning as essential processes by which recovery can occur at the individual level.

Part I Recovery

Early longitudinal research by Ciompi (2005) in Europe, Harding et al. (1987) in the US and others challenged the pessimistic assumption held by many professionals at the time that severe mental illness is long-term and chronic, and that remediation of long-lasting and chronic symptoms coupled with dependency upon mental health services is the best available outcome. Implicit in this traditional conceptual framework was the view of the service user as a passive recipient of specialist medical and social care, with little input from the service users themselves. The importance of these longitudinal studies was to uncover the multiple outcomes associated with severe mental illness and to show that many people did progress beyond a state of merely chronic remediation. Thus the concept of recovery began to obtain legitimacy (Sullivan 1997).

Although there are many perceptions and definitions of recovery, Anthony (1993) developed a definition that many regard as cornerstone:

> [A] deeply personal, unique process of changing one's attitudes, values, feelings, goals, skills and/or roles. It is a way of living

a satisfying, hopeful, and contributing life even with limitations caused by the illness. Recovery involves the development of new meaning and purpose in one's life as one grows beyond the catastrophic effects of mental illness.

Implicit in this view of recovery is a highly individual process of coming to terms with one's own life experience and of redefinition of identity from 'patienthood' to citizenship, a process in which lifelong learning plays a crucial part. A similar point is made by Deegan when she stated that 'any person with severe mental illness can grow beyond the limits imposed by his or her illness' (Deegan 1993). If, as Deegan implies, developmental learning is a core part of the recovery process, then this has major implications for mental health services. One of the necessary and sufficient preconditions of recovery is that it occurs in a context in which the recovering individual is fully included in and able to engage in work and other meaningful activities, and that these are so organised that social inclusion is possible. The experience of mental illness can and usually does profoundly affect the individual's sense of self, of personal identity. In times of crisis, the self can cease to be capable of independent functioning and retreats to being an institutionally or service-defined 'product' or 'entity'. At this point, services capable of 'holding' people when in acute crisis are certainly necessary and indeed essential. Catastrophic events such as involuntary admission negatively affect many areas of life, and many of those who experience mental disorder hope for a return to or recovery of aspects of their life that they had before. Desire for a return of self-confidence, self-esteem and positive hope for the future, coupled with being believed by others to be capable of recovery, help provide an individual with the drive to seek to recover, to learn how to adapt to the challenges they face and to find new ways of 'being in the world'.

Lifelong learning is key to the process of recovery, putting into motion a process in which the person reclaims their 'sense of self', in which the painful episodes and experiences of mental illness form an ensemble around which a new sense of self can grow, a sense of self which is not institutionally or externally defined. To recover, the service user employs existing learning and acquires new learning alongside unlearning, which together form a new identity as someone who has been profoundly influenced by, but who has moved beyond, the traditional mental health service identities of 'patient' or 'client'. The paradox for mental health services is that they themselves are institutions, complex organisational bureaucracies, and it is at the very least challenging for such services to provide the intensely personal and private fulcrum for change that many point to as the essential starting point for recovery.

Recovery from mental illness involves many different factors and is much more than recovery from the illness itself. 'People with mental illness may have to recover from the stigma they have incorporated into their very being; from the iatrogenic effects of treatment settings; from lack of recent opportunities for self-determination; from the negative side effects of unemployment; and from crushed dreams' (Deegan1993). A great deal of new learning is required for different aspects of an individual's recovery in a complex and often lengthy process. Lifelong learning and recovery are in this sense both part of the process of forging a meaningful, coherent pattern out of the disparate and disjointed experiences that are often created through the experience of 'being mentally ill'. Ralph, Kidder and Phillips (2000) concluded that 'recovery can be defined as a process of learning to approach each day's challenges, overcome our disabilities, learn skills, live independently and contribute to society'. According to the European Commission, lifelong learning is 'all learning activity undertaken throughout life, with the aim of improving knowledge, skills and competence, within a personal, civic, social and/or employment-related perspective' (EU COM 2001). Both these approaches are describing lifelong learning and recovery as ways to generate a strengthened locus of control, gains in empowerment and increased independence.

Part I of this book comprises five chapters. Helen Glover starts out with a comprehensive overview of the whole agenda covered in this book from a service-user perspective and explores the possible linkages between recovery, social inclusion, empowerment and lifelong learning. She discusses whether this does, or potentially could, constitute a new paradigm for mental health. She cautions that this might, in certain circumstances, be 'just words' and warns against mental health services badging themselves as 'recovery-oriented' when in reality nothing much may have changed. Chapters 2 and 3 describe two alternative views as to under what conditions recovery can best be fostered and encouraged. In Chapter 2, Wilma Boevink describes her work in the TREE programme (Towards Recovery, Empowerment and Experiential Expertise) at the Trimbos Institute in the Netherlands, an approach driven and led by service users, which sets out to provide effective methods and strategies developed by people with mental health vulnerabilities in order to help themselves as their own programmers of recovery. The TREE programme runs user self-management groups and is staffed by trainers who are themselves service users who pass on their own knowledge and experience to others with respect to mental health difficulties, with the long-term aim of facilitating empowerment in as many ways as they can. Chapter 3 also focuses on a user-led and user-driven approach, but this time located in the voluntary sector in the United Kingdom. Barbara Evans and Kate Sault describe how the Wellness Recovery Action Planning (WRAP) approach, based initially on the American work of Mary Ellen Copeland, has been applied in a European context. Again, this approach is user-driven and puts forward a systematic and structured approach through which service users can self-manage their own difficulties. In Chapter 4, Robert Surber describes his journey from his initial assumption that he could, as a service provider, run, plan and manage recovery for the service user, to the realisation that this was precisely what he could not do – again emphasising that recovery is an intensely personal experience and that perhaps his best contribution as a service provider was to step out of the way and, to put it bluntly, to stop interfering. Boardman and Shepherd, in Chapter 5, describe a model and methodology for the total reconstruction of mental health services so that they might in fact offer the new perspective and direction in order for recovery to happen in practice. This chapter also gives an early indication of how successful this approach can be when actually implemented.

Part II: Social Inclusion and Employment

While social inclusion certainly includes the critically important issue of ensuring that people with mental health difficulties get back to the open employment market, it is also about participation in society in a broader and deeper sense. Social inclusion is about more than access, or improving access to mainstream services. It is about participation in the community, as employees, students, volunteers, teachers, carers, parents, advisors, residents, as active citizens. People with mental health difficulties have a right to access social, economic, educational, recreational and cultural opportunities, as well as physical health services, that are available to the general population. Promoting a social inclusion and employment agenda for those with mental illness is part of the shift of paradigm from a model of care that saw the 'mental patient' as an essentially passive recipient of care, whether delivered by a social worker, nurse, psychiatrist or peer support worker, to a far more active and dynamic partnership model where the service user is not only seen as defining and steering their own care in the community, but also where they are seen, and see themselves, as citizens with human rights.

As a reflection of the importance of these issues, social inclusion policy and legislation against social exclusion have been developed over the last few years both at the European and national levels (MHE 2006). Social exclusion refers to the extent to which individuals are unable to participate in key areas of economic, social and cultural life: 'An individual is socially excluded if he or she does not participate in key activities of the society in which he or she lives' (Burchardt, LeGrand and Piachaud 2002). The major indicators of social exclusion relate to a combination of linked, inter-related problems: unemployment, poor skills, low incomes, poor housing, high crime, poor physical health and family breakdown. Social *inclusion* therefore needs to address all these problems.

Social inclusion and employment in particular are vital issues for those experiencing mental health difficulties. From an ethical viewpoint, the right to work is included in the Universal Declaration of Human Rights (United Nations 1948) and has been incorporated into national legislation such as the UK Disability Discrimination Act 1995 (Crowther et al. 2001), as well as in the social policy and legislation of many other European countries (MHE 2006). If a person with mental illness is in paid employment, then society benefits from the contribution made by the person through their work and also from the reduction or elimination in state aid paid out to the individual. Employment can also bring many advantages for the individual who suffers from mental illness. It can increase the level of financial and social independence, reduce the stigma associated with mental illness, and increase self-esteem and self-worth through, for example, improving his or her social standing within community (Linhorst 2006). Employment can strengthen self-identity because people define themselves, and society defines people, in part by their work (Linhorst 2006). Employment provides a means of structuring life (Rinaldi et al. 2004) and increases lifestyle regularity, both of which can be important in the maintenance of prescription drug schedules. Employment also facilitates greater social interaction and allows people to develop new social relationships. Additionally, it can increase a mentally ill individual's acceptance within society (Kinsey, Hyde and Jackson 2003) and, because employment raises the standard of living of an individual, it provides the individual with an increased range of lifestyle and consumer choices (Linhorst 2006).

Severely mentally ill service users tend in most European societies to have very low levels of employment. Unemployment or poorly paid, temporary jobs have been shown to have a negative impact upon the mental health of the people concerned (STAKES 2000). Two decades or so ago, employment opportunities for people with severe and enduring mental illness were almost completely absent. Ryan et al. (1999) found that 99 per cent of the severely mentally ill were unemployed, and had been so for over three years. Similar findings were made by Burns et al. (1999) and Thornicroft (1998). More recently, Burns et al. (2007) found unemployment levels of 77 per cent amongst those with long-term mental illness in the European study EQOLISE.

In Chapter 6, Davidson, Flanagan and Styron set the agenda for mental health in terms of a radical model of community inclusion, going far beyond the notion of the service user making an optimal adaptation within the confines of mental health services. They empha-sise the important distinction between *integration* and *inclusion*: 'The community inclusion paradigm argues that people with long-term disabilities – including people with long-term *psychiatric* disabilities – should be accepted and welcomed by their communities as they are, with whatever conditions they may have, without having to be cured, fixed, or otherwise made to conform to selected societal norms first'. In Chapter 7, Schneider focuses on the issue of employment as a crucial aspect of social inclusion. She describes the Individual Placement and Support (IPS) model of facilitating employment for those with long-term mental health difficulties and gives an account of implementing such an approach in Nottingham in the UK. Finally in this section in Chapter 8, Greacen and Jouet, using source material drawn from the EMILIA project, describe a methodology for identifying the barriers and obstacles preventing full social inclusion, as well as identifying evidence-based strategies for overcoming these obstacles.

Part III: Empowerment and Lifelong Learning

Empowerment can be seen as the process by which people take control of their own lives and make their own choices, acting where necessary to overcome obstacles preventing that fulfilment. It is about increasing the capacity of individuals to become more in control over their lives and is a means which allows greater participation in decisions, along with increased dignity and respect and a sense of belonging and con-tributing to a wider community. It is important to view empowerment in this broader context, as referring to the level of choice, influence and control which service users can exercise over all events in their life, and about their rights as citizens. This issue is well summarised by WHO (2010). 'The key to empowerment is the removal of formal or informal barriers and the transformation of power relations between individuals, communities, services and governments. Power is central to the idea of empowerment'. With regard to mental health services, empowerment can be seen as referring to the level of choice, influence and control which service users can exercise over services provided. With respect to their experiences of services, it is often the case that they are at a minimum poorly informed, and often poorly consulted and/or poorly treated by mental health service. Historically, people with mental health problems did not have a voice; they and their families were not involved in decision-making processes in policy and practice of mental health services, and they had to face social exclusion and discrimination in all facets of life. Current reports on mental health in the European region show that this has not changed significantly in recent years (WHO 2009). Disempowerment of mental health services users has operated at societal, service provision and individual levels. At the individual level, many service users remain traumatised for long periods of time with damaged internal senses of identity and self-worth through their difficult experience of living in society with a mental illness – a process of internalisation of the external stigma which society itself has traditionally imposed upon them.

For the European Commission (EU COM 2001), lifelong learning is 'learning that is pursued throughout life: learning that is flexible, diverse and continues in many different contexts and settings', with four broad and mutually supportive objectives: personal fulfilment, active citizenship, social inclusion and employability/adaptability. Lifelong learning is considered as an important part of the European Union's Lisbon strategy according to which the European Union aimed to become by 2010, the most competitive and dynamic knowledge-based economic area in the world, as well as a more cohesive and inclusive society. Acquiring and continuously updating and upgrading skills and competences is considered a prerequisite for the personal development of all citizens and for participation in all aspects of society.

Delors (1996) refers to the four 'pillars' of lifelong learning:

- **Learning to know** – learning how to learn rather than specific sets of knowledge
- **Learning to do** – developing the capability to adapt and respond creatively to new challenges and new demands
- **Learning to live together and with others** – peacefully resolving conflict, discovering other people and their cultures, and fostering community capability
- **Learning to be** – learning that contributes to a person's complete development, of mind and body, aesthetic and cultural appreciation, and spirituality

Delors' model shows that there are clearly important links between empowerment and lifelong learning. It views lifelong learning as a central component of a process leading to personal fulfilment, social inclusion, employment in meaningful work activity and a role within society as an active and valued citizen. It is arguable that a significant component of personal fulfilment is both the capacity and the experience of making one's own life choices – the central feature of empowerment. Equally, social inclusion is central, and in this sense, lifelong learning can perhaps best be seen as a core mechanism facilitating for the individual concerned a fully socially inclusive role in society.

In Chapter 9, Ryan, Baumann and Griffiths give an overview of empowerment, both in terms of clarifying a variety of ambiguities surrounding the use of the term and describing its evidence-base. In Chapter 10, Crepaz-Keay, coming from a service-user perspective, gives recommendations for practice and advocates the use of a set of indicators of empowerment, applicable at the national level. In Chapter 11, Anderson and Holmshaw address the issue of empowerment in terms of exploring service-user involvement both as researchers and teachers in the higher education setting. The remaining chapters of the book discuss lifelong learning drawing in different ways upon the experience of the EMILIA project, a recent European project on the role of lifelong learning in the social inclusion of mental health service users. Ogunleye, Griffiths, Dawson and Nybjerg, in Chapter 12, give a broad overview of the meaning and policy context of lifelong learning and outline the health benefits of lifelong learning to disadvantaged groups such as those experiencing long term mental health difficulties. Kaunonen and Ramon in Chapter 13, drawing on qualitative research evidence from the EMILIA project, give an account of organisational mechanisms, such as the Learning Organisation, necessary to promote lifelong learning. The following two chapters describe lifelong learning from a service-user perspective. In Chapter 14, Nilsen gives a powerful account of the barriers, obstacles and difficulties in developing systems and structures which genuinely enable empowerment. In Chapter 15, Nieminen, Nilsen, Vila, Solá and the Fenix user group from Tuzla in Bosnia summarise the service-user perceptions of the benefits of lifelong learning, drawing on data from the Emilia project qualitative research. Finally, in Chapter 16, Stenfors-Hayes and Ryan offer a close analysis of the role of the service-user trainer, which was utilised throughout the lifelong learning programmes in the EMILIA project, describing this role in terms of a pedagogic model of teaching and learning.

The EMILIA project

The EMILIA Project (Empowerment of Mental Health Service Users through Lifelong Learning, Integration and Action), described in several chapters of this book, was a large EU Framework 6 action research project, based in eight demonstration sites across Europe (Athens, Barcelona, Bodø, London, Paris, Tuzla, Warsaw, Zealand) and supported by several other key institutions (Aarhus University, the Karolinska Institute in Stockholm, the Faculty of Social Work at the University of Ljubljana, Middlesex University, Tampere University and the University of Vilnius). The overall aim of the EMILIA Project was to reduce social exclusion in people with serious mental illness through lifelong learning. This included improving the way in which service users could experience greater participation both in service delivery and in education and training, including greater social inclusion in general, through paid employment and significant activities, however locally defined.

Throughout the project, the eight demonstration sites varied considerably in culture, economic situation, the structure of mental health services, as well as in readiness and ability to offer social inclusion and recovery opportunities to people with severe mental illness experience. Seven of the sites were providing mental health services, while one site was a university faculty (London); two of the clinical sites were also research centres (Zealand in Denmark and Warsaw in Poland). Of the seven sites, five had a hospital as the core of their service, and three had community services such as day centres and group homes (Athens, Greece), a user group (Tuzla, Bosnia) and an out-patient clinic (Zealand).

The focus of the EMILIA project on enhancing social inclusion and recovery for people with long-term mental illness called for a process of adaptation in the demonstration sites, given that meeting these objectives required an organisational structure and a local social context that not only welcomed service users but also was ready to offer them opportunities far beyond those usually on offer in clinical practice in preparing them for a more independent life, employment and enhancing their social network as means of empowerment (Ramon, Ryan and Urek 2010, Ramon 2011).

The project, funded by the EU under its Framework 6 from 2005 to 2010, recruited adults (aged 18 and above), diagnosed as having severe and enduring mental illness (schizophrenia and bipolar disorder), in contact with mental health services for at least three years and who were not in paid employment. They were offered a series of training modules with other service users, and opportunities for employment or significant activities within the demonstration sites as well as connecting them to potential employers outside the sites in which the project operated.

An extensive quantitative and qualitative evaluation took place at all demonstration sites at baseline, ten months and twenty months in terms of their socio-demographic status, their take up of the training and of unpaid and paid employment, their own evaluation of the impact of participation in the project in relation to employment, social interaction, training activities, opportunities and obstacles, and goals for the near future, as well as related organisational changes in the demonstration sites. The project in many ways succeeded in creating user employment and supported pathways both within demonstration site organisations and in competitive employment.

The final report of the EMILIA Project can be consulted at http://www.mdx. ac.uk/Assets/3a(i)1%20EMILIA%20FINAL%20PUBLISHABLE10610FIN3_ predit.pdf.

References

Anthony, W. A. (1993). 'Recovery from Mental Illness: The Guiding Vision of the Mental Health Service System in the 1990s', *Psychosocial Rehabilitation Journal*, XVI(4), 11–23.

Barnes, M. and Bowl, R. (2000). *Taking over the Asylum – Empowerment and Mental Health* (Basingstoke: Palgrave Macmillan).

Burchardt, T., LeGrand, J. and Piachaud, D. (2002). 'Degrees of Exclusion: Developing a Dynamic, Multidimensional Measure', in J. Hills, J. LeGrand and D. Piachaud (eds). *Understanding Social Exclusion* (Oxford: Oxford University Press).

Burns, T., Creed, F., Fahy, T., Thompson, S., Tyrer, P. and White, I. (1999). 'Intensive versus Standard Case Management for Severe Psychotic Illness: A Randomised Trial', *Lancet*, CCCLII, 2185–9.

Burns, T., Catty, J., Becker, J., Drake, R. E., Fioritti, A., Knapp, M. et al. (2007). 'The Effectiveness of Supported Employment for People with Severe Mental Illness: A Randomised Controlled Trial', *Lancet*, CCCLXX, 1146–52.

Ciompi, L. (2005). 'The Natural History of Schizophrenia in the Long Term', In L. Davidson, C. M. Harding and L. Spaniol (eds). *Recovery from Severe Mental Illness: Research Evidence and Implications for Practice* (Boston: University of Boston), 224–35.

Crowther, R. E., Marshall, M, Bond, G. R. and Huxley, P. (2001). 'Helping People with Severe Mental Illness to Obtain Work: Systematic Review', *British Medical Journal*, CCCXXII, 204–8.

Deegan, P. E. (1993). 'Recovering Our Sense of Value after Being Labeled Mentally Ill', *Journal of Psychosocial Nursing and Mental Health Services*, XXXI, 7–11.

Delors, J. (1996). *Learning: the Treasure Within* (Paris: UNESCO).

EU COM (2001). 'Making a European Area of Life Long Learning. 678 Final'. Brussels: Commission of the European Communities, http://eur-lex.europa. eu/LexUriServ/LexUriServ.do?uri=COM:2001:0678:FIN:EN:PDF, date accessed 15 December 2011.

Harding, C. M., Brooks, G. W., Ashikaga, T., Strauss, J. S. and Breier, A. (1987). 'The Vermont Longitudinal Study of Persons with Severe Mental Illness', *American Journal of Psychiatry*, CXLIV, 718–26.

Kinsey, M. B., Hyde, P. S. and Jackson, E. (2003). 'Involvement of State and Local Mental Health Authorities in Addressing the Employment Needs of People with Serious Mental Illness', in D. P. Moxley and J. R. Finch (eds). *Sourcebook of Rehabilitation and Mental Health Practice* (New York: Kluwer Academic/Plenum Publishers).

Linhorst, D. M. (2006). *Empowering People with Severe Mental Illness: A Practical Guide* (Oxford: Oxford University Press).

Mental Health Europe (MHE) (2008). 'From Exclusion to Inclusion – The Way Forward to Promoting Social Inclusion of People with Mental Health Problems in Europe', http://www.mhe-sme.org/assets/files/From%20Exclusion%20to%20Inclusion-Final%20version.pdf, date accessed 14 December 2011.

Ralph, R. O., Kidder, K. and Phillips, D. (2000). 'Can We Measure Recovery? A Compendium of Recovery and Recovery-Related Instruments', *The Evaluation Center@HSRI*, www.hsri.org/eval/eval.html, date accessed 14 June 2011.

Ramon, S., Ryan, P. and Urek, M. (2010), 'Attempting to Mainstream Ethnicity in a Multi-Country EU Mental Health and Social Inclusion Project: Lessons for Social Work', *European Journal of Social Work*, XIII, 2, 163–82.

Ramon, S. (2011) 'Organisational change in the context of recovery-oriented services', *Journal of Mental Health Training, Education and Practice*, The, 6, 1, 38–46.

Repper, J. and Perkins, R. (2003). *Social Inclusion and Recovery: A Model for Mental Health Practice* (Baillere Tindall).

Rinaldi, M., Mcneil, K., Firn, M., Koletsi, M., Perkins, R. and Singh, S. P. (2004). 'What are the Benefits of Evidence-Based Supported Employment for Patients with First-Episode Psychosis?', *Psychiatric Bulletin*, XXVIII, 281–4.

Ryan, P., Ford, R., Beadsmoore, A. and Muijen, M. (1999). 'The Enduring Relevance of Case Management', *BJ Social Work*, XXIX, 97–125.

Slade, M. (2009). *Personal Recovery and Mental Illness: A Guide for Mental Health Professionals* (Cambridge: Cambridge Medical).

STAKES (2000). Public Health Approach on Mental Health in Europe. National Research and Development Centre for Mental Health: Helsinki, http://groups.stakes.fi/NR/rdonlyres/1EB54ED4-EC61-405A-8DF5-5B7829917069/0/public2.pdf, date accessed 14 December 2011.

Sullivan, W. P. (1997). 'A Long and Winding Road: The Process of Recovery from Severe Mental Illness', in L. Spaniol, C. Gagne and M. Koehler (eds). *Psychological and Social Aspects of Psychiatric Disability* (Boston: Center for Psychiatric Rehabilitation).

Thornicroft, G. (1998). 'The PRiSM Psychosis Study articles 1–10', *British Journal of Psychiatry*, CLXIII, 363–431.

United Nations (1948). Universal Declaration of Human Rights, New York: UN.

WHO Regional Office for Europe (2009). 'Policies and Practices for Mental Health in Europe – Meeting the challenges', Copenhagen: WHO Regional Office for Europe.

WHO Regional Office for Europe (2010), 'User Empowerment in Mental Health', Copenhagen: WHO Regional Office for Europe. http://www.euro.who.int/__data/assets/pdf_file/0020/113834/E93430.pdf, date accessed 14 December 2011.

Part I
Recovery

1
Recovery, Lifelong Learning, Empowerment and Social Inclusion: Is a New Paradigm Emerging?

Helen Glover

My experience of mental illness has given me far more than it has dared to take away. In essence, my journey has given me an opportunity to learn and thrive. I lost my way for some time during the years of seeking help. Despite good intentions, I was inadvertently invited to ultimately believe that 'others', whether they were family, friends or mental health professionals, were my experts and that they were the only people who could get my life back on track. I have learnt since, that it is nearly impossible to reclaim a sense of citizenship and personal recovery from the position of seeing 'others' as being the 'expert' of your own life. Now, as a mental health professional, the wisdom of lived experience challenges me to be ever mindful of the fact that:

> *[we] cannot recover people – but we can get in the way of people in their own efforts of recovery.*
> *We cannot empower people – but we can utilise our power to dis-empower others.*
> *We cannot create a person's sense of citizenship but we can offer programs and services that reinforce a person's sense of 'illness-ship'.*
> *We cannot teach people to have hope or rediscover themselves, but we can inadvertently inhibit a person's sense of discovery and learning.*
> *Our responsibility is not to assess, manage, monitor, teach and rehabilitate, but to create environments where a person can recognise their own mastery, and continue to learn and thrive beyond the limitations invited by the experience of mental illness or distress.*

This chapter poses a very important question. Is a new paradigm of practice emerging regarding how people who experience mental illness or distress are supported to reclaim a life beyond the impacts of mental illness? Is it possible for support and treatment to move beyond the sole focus of providing relief from distress and adopt a focus centred on personal recovery, underpinned by empowerment, social connectedness and lifelong learning?

The promise of a new paradigm that centres itself on citizenship and personal recovery is what people with a lived experience and mental health advocates have been demanding for what 'feels like an eternity'. The mental health service reform and transformation agendas of many countries, such as the United States (SAMHSA 2010), the United Kingdom, parts of Europe (European Union 2010), New Zealand (Mental Health Commission 2009) and Australia (Australian Government 2010) are starting to articulate within their policy direction the need to provide services that more directly focus on recovery, empowerment, social inclusion and lifelong learning.

Aligning to this new paradigm is not simple and will challenge the very heart and existing foundation that services have been built upon. It will require mental health services and practitioners to provide support and treatment environments that no longer focus on illness management alone. Creating environments of support that are more fully aligned to supporting a person's appreciation of their self-mastery over distress, while remaining connected to their life direction, and outside the context of an illness experience will be called for. Ultimately, appreciating that supporting personal recovery will require a transformative (Taylor 2008) learning platform as opposed to a treatment and service environment is an essential shift for both policy and services to embrace. This approach will fundamentally transform the nature of service delivery and cannot but help increase the relevance of mental health support to peoples' lives.

Change the person or the service?

It is encouraging and extremely refreshing that the attention on who and what needs to change is slowly starting to shift away from the person who may experience mental illness or distress to the systems of care that provide support and treatment. This change in focus is somewhat radical and difficult for systems of care to maintain, as historically they have been held responsible for managing the care and treatment of people who experience mental illness and distress. It is tempting for systems of care to revert their focus to assessing, fixing, treating, managing, monitoring, empowering, motivating and recovering the person as opposed to remaining vigilant about transforming and reforming service environments. Often, systems of care will blame the person for not engaging in their support and treatment options, rather than enquiring what is it about the service environs and processes that a person does not find useful, or finds difficult to engage with.

New paradigm or old paradigm dressed in 'sheep's clothing'?

Mental health services can create an illusion that they are transforming how they deliver services by using the language of recovery at a superficial level, yet still remain entrenched in practices centred on changing the person. Understandably, people feel a level of cynicism and disappointment when they experience a misalignment between what is upheld and promised in policy and what they actually experience in practice.

In Australia, and this may also be true for many other countries, it is unlikely that a modern mental health service exists that has not rebadged their service framework and programmes towards a recovery and social inclusion agenda, with a focus on empowerment and lifelong learning. While this is greatly encouraging, questions need to be asked as to whether the renaming of service culture has really altered the traditional care and protection ideology and practice that have been, and are presently, core to most mental health service provision. This question is equally applicable to both clinical services and community support agencies. There is a real risk that the existing paradigm, with its emphasis on managed care, expert determination, monitoring and risk aversion, will remain dominant and the promise of a new paradigm will be experienced solely as 'buzz-words' and rebadging, if policy, service culture and practice cannot be realigned. Even the potential impact of the term 'paradigm shift', in its over-use and misuse, has weakened its ability to communicate the magnitude of the shift required. Just to rebadge existing practices and frameworks with new language alone may not only poorly serve new ways of being, but may even strengthen existing practices and processes, providing an illusion that a shift has taken place, where in reality services remain dominant and in control of peoples' lives. For a new paradigm to be fully realised, it must be enshrined in policy, evident in practice and ultimately experienced by people who access services.

Some services have, for example, renamed their 'care plans' to 'individual recovery plans'. However, the processes underpinning these so-called recovery plans remain unchanged. They remain instigated, formulated, managed and monitored by mental health workers, kept in organisational files within locked cabinets, far away from being usable by the persons themselves in their own self-direction and self-management. Getting a signature on the plan and providing a copy to the person in no way speaks to supporting a person in their recovery, inclusion, learning or empowerment!

Thomas Kuhn (1962) used the term 'paradigm', within the scientific community to simply mean a collection of shared understanding or beliefs regarding a certain topic, or a set of agreements concerning how a problem can be understood or responded to. We tend to refute or ignore evidence that lies outside any dominant paradigms, thereby giving more credibility to the existing paradigm. Zucconi (2008) articulates that a genuine paradigm shift occurs only when the current way of understanding or responding to a problem is considered to be no longer useful or valid. A new paradigm emerges when the old ways of thinking or responding are surrendered to new ways of thinking and responding that are thought to be better. It is difficult, if not impossible, for a new paradigm to hold on to existing ways as well as adopt new ways.

Shifting core beliefs

Historically, some of the shared thinking and beliefs about people who experience a mental illness have not been aligned to the concept that people can and do reclaim a life beyond services and a life beyond illness. Core beliefs about the nature of mental illness have not shifted greatly. Despite people with a lived experience demanding that mental health services change their ways, many of the institutionalised beliefs and practices still remain current and dominant. Although many of these beliefs have no firm foundation and truth, their mythology remains active and has left a legacy that plays out in the modern context of providing care. Table 1.1 highlights the unquestioned and entrenched nature of these historically based core beliefs as they reposition themselves within the daily routines in current practices. A new paradigm would need to seriously challenge their currency and relevance to the provision of helpful support, as determined by the expertise from lived experience informants.

Table 1.1 Historical beliefs influencing current practice

Historical belief	Corresponding examples of contemporary mental health practice
People who experience a mental illness	
Will be permanently unwell	• Case management • Long-term care arrangements • Group/hostel supported housing arrangements • Individual funding based on a permanent need • Encouragement to let go of roles and responsibilities – for example, work, study, parenting • Support to access permanent Disability Benefit Entitlements
Will need increasing amounts of support over time	• Increase number of services funded to manage people in the community. • Increase in the number of services in a person's life. • Permanent and individualised funding packages
Cannot take responsibility and will require management by others	• Care-planning processes undertaken by services without the person's involvement • Decisions being made by 'others' • Monitoring undertaken as the responsibility of services • Compliance driven • Services providing a whole-of-life response to people • Service providers working to attain people's personal goals and desires
Are at risk to themselves or others	• Risk assessment determined by 'others' • Risk management plans created and monitored by 'others' • No involvement or expectation of a person participating in managing their risky behaviour • No evidence of shared responsibility and partnerships with the person • Overuse of the Mental Health Act • Hospital admission as an only response to crisis situations • Mental Health Act status seen as an admission and discharge criteria
Require professional help in order to recover	• Service to service referral • No consideration of self as a support strategy • No consideration of the benefits of natural or community responses before or in lieu of a mental health service response

(*continued*)

20

Table 1.1   Continued

Historical belief	Corresponding examples of contemporary mental health practice
People who experience a mental illness	
	• Dominance of paid professionals and workers in people's lives
'Lack Insight' and cannot make meaning of their distress or experiences	• Psychoeducation groups and programmes • Others make meaning of the person's experience without their input • Refute personal meaning that differs from the dominant understanding as 'in-sightless' • Documentation solely undertaken by 'others' • Reviews and planning activities not directed by the person but by the service team
Need a stress-free environment free from social responsibilities	• Provision of permanent social benefits and disability supports • Low stimulation environments within treatment settings • Service activities not linked to real life situations (craft, outings)
Are burdensome and detract from the quality of life	• 'Carer's pension' • Respite for carers programmes • Disability support pension/benefits • Low expectation environments • Rewards to workers for working with 'difficult' people
Will need to be rehabilitated back into the community	• Structured residential and non-residential programmes to learn living skills • Support packages, including housing and set-up funds, create a 'service environment' in individuals' homes, but are seen as 'living in the community'
Cannot build relationships	• Services provide 'un-natural' social environments, which are illness saturated. To access the service, individuals must wear their mental illness on their sleeve; these facilities are not open to the general public. • Services create unnatural 'social' environments by supporting individuals to access shopping centres and coffee shops; there is limited access to meaningful social interaction
Have difficulty motivating themselves	• Individuals are labelled as 'not motivated' when they do not want to engage in pre-planned activities they are not interested in

Do services enable or inadvertently disable people?

The principle of 'do no harm' underpins both medical and social service responses to people. The notion of 'do no harm' implies that there is a capacity of both services and those that provide help to harm others. Unfortunately, it is rare for a person to recount their experience of mental illness without identifying and experiencing a number of other losses and treatment trauma. Sadly, there is so much more that a person has to reclaim than simply overcoming symptoms of a mental illness. What emerges from these narratives are disturbingly reoccurring themes (Deegan 1988, Johnstone 2000, Onken et al. 2002, Jeffs 2010, Hertfordshire Partnership Foundation NHS Trust 2008, Scottish Recovery Network 2008). These recurring themes have little to do with the symptoms of illness, but relate more to how systems inadvertently disable processes of recovery and citizenship. This discussion would be incomplete if it remained silent on the critical need to renegotiate issues of power relations, stigma and institutionalisation within a new paradigm. In receiving assistance, there is an added risk that mental health services may disconnect a person from a real and ordinary life and invite them into their 'illness-ship' as part of their 'package deal'. Barrett (1998) paints a sad picture of the 'modern schizophrenic', living on 'the outer edge of personhood, trapped between the poles of sickness and health in anticipation of a return to the community of the healthy that is not forthcoming'. Estroff (1993), a passionate voice championing change within psychiatric structures, has repeatedly argued that it is mental health services themselves that entrap and stigmatise people and support them to become 'full time crazy people'. Myers (2010, p. 503) in support, argues that it is extremely difficult, if not impossible, for people to escape from such environments, when they are asked to 'subsist on meagre government benefits, take advantage of social services, compliantly accept medications despite severe side effects, keep to themselves and obey their case managers'. The illness experience has become somewhat 'privileged and institutionalised'.

The disabling factors often associated with mental illnesses such as schizophrenia, may have less to do with actual symptomatology, than with the experiences of loss of hope, expectation and opportunities that 'helping' environments inadvertently invite people to participate within.

Questions have been raised from within the psychiatric profession (Summerfield 2001; Tsao, Tummala and Roberts 2008) as to whether the provision of mental healthcare itself is a contributing factor to a person's sense of institutionalisation and stigma. Sartorius (2002) goes even further in suggesting that professionally induced stigma could be considered as iatrogenic, resulting from the medical process itself, but limits the naming of such practices to the impact of labelling, side effects of treatments and attitudes held by mental health practitioners. Iatrogenic injury or illness, caused as a result of health or medical intervention, has usually been associated with error or misjudgement, but not connected to the day-to-day service structures and processes common to mental health service provision.

When mental health services intentionally create treatment and support environments that ultimately reinforce a sense of inability, disability, disconnection and institutionalisation, then those practices must be highlighted and shamed as iatrogenic. There probably is no greater iatrogenic injury than this, yet many of the practices that contribute to such iatrogenic injury are still upheld as 'best practice'. The evidence of such iatrogenic practice is extensive and permeates many narratives as disabling peoples' ability to reclaim a full life. Simply put, these experiences are socially constructed, detrimental and unnecessarily impact on a person's ability to reclaim a life beyond mental illness. Griffiths and Ryan (2008), in discussing the connection between recovery and lifelong learning, name the need to overcome iatrogenic service environments as a common part of the recovery processes, stressing the importance of adopting a lifelong learning approach to equip someone to do this. It is somewhat ironic and outrageous that mental health services should be supporting people in lifelong learning processes to manage the injuries and trauma that have been iatrogenically induced.

Some of the numerous loss and trauma-related injuries that people have associated with the experience and treatment of a mental illness are highlighted in Table 1.2.

These messages can no longer be ignored and classified as subjective or inconsequential. There is an urgent and pressing need to address these common service practices that inadvertently lock someone out of their own life and promote service providers to be 'agents of control'.

Shifting from clinically to personally informed recovery

The wisdom of people who have found a way to reclaim a life beyond the impact of mental illness, has many insights to offer a new paradigm of practice. Their many narratives constantly attest to peoples' ability to self-right over adversity and defy negative prognoses given by mental health professionals as their capacity to resume a quality of life.

Table 1.2 Potential negative impacts of treatment and social environments for people who experience mental illness

Impacts from treatment and support environments
- impact of incarceration, hospitalisation, forced treatment
- impact of medication and side effects
- experience of treatment as trauma
- participation in low or non-stimulating environments
- participation in illness saturated environments
- impact of professional discrimination, and prejudices
- loss of identity through institutionalisation processes
- loss of autonomy
- reinforcement of recipiency role
- loss of power and control and impacts of others' control and power
- non-welcoming environments

Impacts from social environment
- loss of roles, work roles, family roles
- lack of opportunities to reclaim work, study
- loss of connection with friends and family
- loss of income, loss of housing
- loss of opportunities to contribute to community and relationships
- lack of access to participate
- non-welcoming environments
- loss of personal resources
- impact of community stigma and prejudices
- impact of self-stigma

The construct of recovery is often confused by services and workers, with many interpreting it through a more 'clinical' gaze than upholding the internal process essential to 'personal' recovery. Although differing, clinical and personal recovery focuses are not in competition with each other; they are often spoken and written as one entity. 'Clinical' recovery focuses on the destination and successful attainment of health-related outcomes, whereas 'personal recovery' recognises the process and self-applied efforts and learning as important. Ideally a person would desire both; one without the other remains incomplete.

Repeated qualitative and quantitative studies (Onken et al. 2002; Harding et al. 1987; Sullivan 1994; Tooth, Kalyanasundarm and Glover 2003; Topor 2001) and many personal narratives have been able to identify some of these essential and common personal efforts required to self-right. These tend not to vary between the nature of illnesses or life adversities that people have overcome. Tooth, Kalyanasundarm and Glover (2003), in a qualitative study of the 'consumer' perspective on recovery from schizophrenia, identified 111 factors that 57 people named as significant in their journey of recovery. It is interesting to note that the factors frequently reported differed somewhat from what professionals often name as important to peoples' recovery. People with a lived experience tended to highlight their internal agency over the external application of support as being significant, such as finding self-determination, self-managing and taking personal responsibility. Furthermore, those in recovery did not appreciate some of the aspects of care that services usually name as helpful, such as medication, hospitalisation and professional help.

Providing a platform for lifelong learning

A person cannot reclaim a life beyond illness and experience well-being in a vacuum of ongoing learning and discovery. The ability to learn from, reflect upon, make sense of and create meaning leading to new action is the essence of personal recovery. The notion of 'well-being' has increasingly entered the mental health arena, providing guidance to a recovery-oriented paradigm, encouraging a shift from a treatment response to a provision of learning platform.

The notion of well-being is not the absence of illness, nor does it emerge through the reduction and eradication of symptoms alone. Mental health has been defined by the World Health Organisation (2011) as 'a state of being where an individual realises their own potential, can cope with the normal stressors of life, can work productively and fruitfully, and is able to make contribution to his or her community'.

It is less about the presence of distress that symptoms and treatment may bring but our mastery over them that is important to recovery. Having a focus of living 'in recovery' (Davidson 2003) as opposed to 'recovering from' invites a lifelong learning process of recognising and appreciating shifts, especially the person's own agency in creating and sustaining such shifts. In an ordinary day in any mental health service, upholding a person's authorship is extremely difficult, let alone supporting and enhancing their meaning-making capacity. Service structures stress the importance of expert and professionally determined assessments, documentation, reviews, handovers and planning processes with little options for them to be shaped, informed and directed by the person seeking help. Such everyday practices may inadvertently reinforce and endorse to a person their illness authorship and identity. Within the ordinariness and routines of everyday work practices of mental health service provision, a person must be offered vital and ongoing opportunities to reshape their authorship and self-directed learning towards well-being and mastery, if the potential of a new paradigm is to be fully realised.

Psycho-education programmes have been the attempt by many service structures to help people diagnosed with a mental illness to learn to manage their illness. Unfortunately, most of these programmes are centred on teaching about the illness experience and its management requirements, with vain hopes that people will become more compliant and adopt lifestyles that are deemed more 'appropriate and healthy'. Such programmes, in their attempts to orchestrate lifelong learning, fail the basic premise that learning is a self-directed and ongoing process that does not occur solely within '8-week' structured courses. Psycho-education at best has equipped people and their families to become experts on illness, as determined by others, and taught prescriptive ways of living life that may not connect with self-expertise, direction and mastery.

A lifelong learning approach within a new paradigm would seek to provide a transformative learning platform that acknowledges its ongoing, self-directed nature, and that true learning does not come easily and without struggle and discomfort. It would acknowledge that a person's discovery already exists within and cannot be provided by another.

To enable and not disable a sense of personal discovery, workers need to utilise their therapeutic relationship and skills to acknowledge that personal learning and shifts are forever taking place, invite reflection, dialogue and debate with the person and be prepared to alter their own understanding and perceptions based on the wisdom from those to whom they offer support. Therefore a new paradigm requires providers to go beyond the monitoring and responding to 'illness' as its core business, but be in relationships with people inviting them to connect to their ongoing learning and personal agency between

1. The permanency of distress – an ability to influence distress (Hope – Despair)
2. Seeing that change comes through the efforts of others – recognising and appreciating the role of self in creating shifts (Active sense of self – Passive sense of self)
3. Resting in others' management and care – negotiating self-management and mastery (Ability to respond – Inability to respond)
4. Accepting others' interpretation and determination alone – reflecting and undertaking self-learning and meaning-making (Discovery – Alienation)
5. Participating in roles that reinforce institutionalisation and illness-ship – participating through a sense of citizenship and full community membership (Connectedness – Disconnectedness).

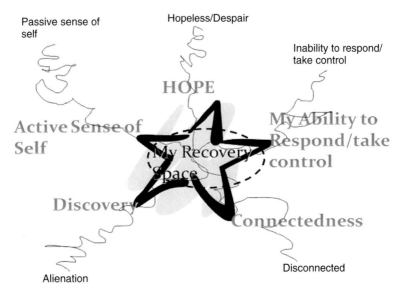

Passive sense of
self

Hopeless/Despair

Inability to respond/
take control

HOPE

Active Sense of
Self

My Ability to
Respond/take
control

My Recovery
Space

Discovery

Connectedness

Alienation

Disconnected

Figure 1.1   Star of Recovery

As a consultant and training facilitator, I saw the need to create a number of constructs that could assist services reconfigure new care frameworks. One of the constructs that underpin a recovery orientation, the *Star of Recovery* (Glover 2007), reflects the above dichotomies through five points: (i) Hope, (ii) Active Sense of Self, (iii) Ability to Respond, (iv) Discovery and (v) Connectedness (see Figure 1.1).

The Star of Recovery is not designed to tempt workers to 'shift' a person from one polarity to the other. The recognition that these polarities are already in existence is important, and services therefore should provide opportunities that enable and not hinder a person's capacity to negotiate between each of these polarities. The five polarities reflect the efforts and processes that people with a lived experience identify as important and essential to self-righting processes.

Empowerment: Renegotiating power from you to me

The shift from external determination to the internal realisation is undoubtedly the major repositioning work that mental health services and providers need to commit to if a new paradigm is to be fully realised. In principle this sounds easy, yet it has proven difficult for many services and providers to let go of their expert manager roles in the lives of others. Maybe one of the reasons is that mental healthcare has increasingly acquired society's authority to 'explain, categorise, treat, detain and prognose' (Summerfield 2001), making it extremely difficult, if not impossible, to let go of the dominant expert position in the lives of others.

This criticism of others positioning themselves as experts extends beyond just rigid biomedical approaches, but to all services that provide responses to people experiencing mental illness or distress. Myers (2010) challenges psychosocial support organisations which traditionally name their approaches as 'recovery-oriented' and 'empowering', that they too may be responsible for denying a person their rightful autonomy.

> It is not easy to let go of the false (but comforting) certainties of traditional mental health – for example, that staff are the true experts (certainly not Consumers) on what is best.
>
> (Myers 2010)

Thankfully, it is not just those with a lived expertise who are advocating for a shift in power. As one professional states:

> People cannot progress in their recovery while others are in control of their lives, so clinicians may need to think how to 'let go' a bit. We may need to share authority and power, have a greater openness to what patients say and wish, and be more trusting and supportive of their personal priorities. Recovery-oriented services will see a shift in our role towards becoming coach, mentor, educator and facilitator.
>
> (Roberts 2007)

Many mental health services and providers believe that their work is to 'empower' others who they perceive as lacking in power and direction. This is not possible, nor helpful. We cannot empower people – we can only *dis*empower them by hindering their natural self-power, autonomy and direction to be exercised. A sense of personal empowerment can only be realised and appreciated as an internal shift. A simple way to remember this is to switch the first two letters of the word **EM**-POWER and create **ME**–POWER.

Services have interpreted this new way of support as having to get people to achieve goals, be motivated, get independent, move from one accomplishment to the next, if they are to justify to funders that as services they are relevant and effective in people's lives. Sadly, it is not uncommon to hear that people will be 'exited' from treatment or support programmes, as they are not achieving or changing fast enough to justify the input of service's valuable resources.

Could services' attempts at social inclusion result in social exclusion?

The experience of institutionalisation, once regarded as a condition resulting from long-stay hospital admissions, has the potential to exist within our current community contexts, and requires re-examining within a new paradigm. With the closure of major psychiatric hospitals came an expectation that the experience of institutionalisation would also be relegated to the history books. This has not been so. Despite most mental health services being provided within the community, institutionalised support approaches are still evident if not prolific.

Programmes that promote social inclusion and tackle social exclusion are thought to assist people to reclaim their relationships and rightful place in the community. These programmes are currently in favour with many government-funding programmes. The challenge is to ensure that in the execution of such programmes mental health services do not reinforce social exclusion. Questions need to be asked as to why mental health services see the need to create specialised programmes for people to meet their non-mental health needs such as relationships, recreation, fitness, general health, education, employment, accommodation and finances through direct mental health pathways. Psychiatric hospitals provided a whole-of-life service and it seems that community-based mental health services are increasingly inheriting the same legacy.

Many mental health services are attempting to become the initial and sole response to people's social, physical, emotional and spiritual needs, but in the process inadvertently create artificial and stigmatising opportunities for people, and erode capacity for people to stay connected to natural networks and real community opportunities. Day centres and drop-in centres provide an illusion of social connection, but tend to reinforce the beliefs that full community membership and associated expectations are unsafe and no longer tenable for their participants. If a core belief of services and funders is that people with a mental illness are fundamentally flawed, then artificial and institutionalised pathways will continue to proliferate.

There are two major considerations for a service committed to supporting connectedness and community membership. It should first consider the natural environments of self-direction, natural relationships and generic community initiatives available to all, prior to instigating any service support response. Second, any service response should be considered artificial and temporary and delivered in a manner whereby the natural connections to self, relationships and community are restored and the artificial support structures can safely be disengaged.

Testing socially inclusive service environs

There are ways to test whether a support initiative is illness-saturated. To answer positively to the following questions indicates that the support provided is institutionally focussed and is a contributor to a person's sense of difference and stigma.

1. Is it difficult for someone without an identity of illness to participate in the same initiative?
2. Does the support or activity require a person to identify with their illness/client-hood in order to participate?
3. Is the support activity a substitute or replication of something already available to community members?
4. Does the support structure or activity advertise or have the image of a worker–client relationship (for example, name badges, uniforms, cars with logos)?
5. Does the support provided connect people to artificial relationships?
6. Is the support provided in a way or time that tells others they do not hold socially valued roles?
   Example: holding a service barbeque for 20 adults during lunchtime on a Thursday would indicate to a passer-by that the members of this group are probably a special needs group as most adults who work do not have barbeques at lunchtime on Thursdays in groups of 20.

A recent story highlights how existing practices can be reshaped to enable inclusion and citizenship, and not reinforce exclusion and institutionalisation.

A support worker, working in a large community-based organisation, was hearing that a number of people wanted to learn meditation techniques as part of their self-management. The quick and nasty service-centric way would be for the service to establish a meditation group, run by this worker, as she also was a trained meditation teacher. She resisted this as she had had her own experience of institutionalised environments and knew that this would not be helpful. She had ascertained from those to whom she provided support that it was unlikely at this point in their recovery that they would participate in a publicly available meditation course. There was a new middle ground to be discovered.

Instead she negotiated with her manager to utilise the programme's resources to run a meditation group for the community, in the local community centre, in which she would support a few interested clients to participate. She advertised the eight-week meditation course in the local paper, with no service insignia attached. The service was in its rightful place as a silent but supportive partner. Twelve members of the community participated of which four were clients of the mental health service. Initially none of the twelve participants knew each other.

She had created an opportunity for a few people who accessed the service to meet their needs in learning different self-management skills, without having to identify that they had an illness or were part of the service. The outcome for many in the group was that new relationships and friendships emerged, and they discovered that it is not just people with a mental illness that experience the stressors of life. This may never have been known if an illness-saturated meditation group was the solution created by the service, just for clients of the service.

Reconsidering Kuhn's (1962) thoughts that an emerging paradigm only emerges when aspects of the existing paradigm are no longer valid or useful leads us to question what mental health services are prepared to give up in order to support a new paradigm. While there is a growing acceptance of a recovery-oriented vision by mental health services, there may be greater challenges in appreciating what is required to foster environments that enable a paradigm shift away from the role of managing a person's care and treatment to that of supporting self-management and mastery. Many mental health services, despite their articulation around a recovery orientation, still see that their core business remains to assess mental status, alleviate symptoms of distress, medicate, risk manage, monitor, review, plan, document, manage care, refer where necessary and rehabilitate into the community. In this position, services have still seated themselves at the head of table as experts and the managers of peoples' lives. The transformation being asked of systems, workers, families, society and people themselves is great, and what will be required for this transformation to be fully realised cannot be underestimated. Just like individuals and families that may need some introduction to these concepts, workers within systems of care will also need support, time and space to integrate policy into practice. Just like an individual journey of recovery, this process for workers and services will also be non-linear and full of rich learning.

To hold space for a new paradigm to fully emerge will be uncomfortable, and from time to time systems of care will lose sight of their intent and retreat to what is more known – familiar ways within the existing paradigm. To not be seduced into this lull, services will require a constant vigil on questioning and testing whether the way in which services are being provided ultimately enable or disable people's ability to reclaim a full life outside the context of illness and service responses. Table 1.3, the Star of Recovery Test Questions (Glover 2009), provides a range of testing questions that may assist service providers to determine the nature of their service invitation.

So the question remains, is a new paradigm emerging? Maybe that question needs to remain unanswered, but constantly raised and revisited. We will only know whether the paradigm of practice is relevant and effective if service systems and practitioners constantly seek out the wisdom of those who know – people who have a lived expertise of overcoming mental illness.

Einstein (1879–1955) provides us with two closing thoughts to help us in our refocus, especially when our energy wanes and we start to doubt our intent of creating new ways of relating to and supporting people to reclaim a life beyond the experience of mental illness and distress:

> We can't solve problems by using the same kind of thinking we used when we created them.
>
> (Einstein, quoted in Calaprice 2005)

and

> Any intelligent fool can make things bigger, more complex, and more violent. It takes a touch of genius – and a lot of courage – to move in the opposite direction.
>
> (Einstein, quoted in Calaprice 2005)

32

Table 1.3 Testing service environments' enabling ability: the Star of Recovery Test Questions

Hope – Despair	
Does my practice infer a permanency of illness or distress?	✗
Have I enquired as to what is important to the person?	✓
Have I enquired as to the hopes and dreams a person has?	✓
Have I been curious about the exceptions to their distress?	✓
Have I been curious as to how the illness experience does not stop a person achieving?	✓
Active sense of self – Passive sense of self	
Have I looked for the initiative that a person is utilising to meet their needs?	✓
Am I assuming that a person is totally stuck and without initiative?	✗
Have I been curious as to how a person is meeting his/her own needs?	✓
Does my support or intervention inadvertently stop the 'self-righting' of the person?	✗
Does my support or intervention invite someone's awareness of their active self (for example, their determination, courage or stubbornness)?	✓
Does a person know more about themselves as their own change agent as a result of my intervention or support?	✓
Does a person know more about 'others' as being their change agent through the support I/we provide?	✗
Personal control and responsibility – Others' control and responsibility	
Have I enquired as to what gets in the way of a person being able to maintain control?	✓
Does the intervention or care I provide infer to the person that they are not in control?	✗
Have I been curious as to what the person remains in control of, despite the distress that they are experiencing?	✓
Am I upholding a client's choice alone without negotiating support?	✗
Have I negotiated the support with the person and their family?	✓
Is there a clear indication of when the current level of support will no longer be required? Does the person have the same understanding?	✓

(*continued*)

Table 1.3 Continued

Discovery – Alienation	
Have I checked for self-meaning?	✓
Have I interpreted the situation and provided an external meaning?	✗
Am I directing the care based on my knowledge of the person's illness?	✗
Am I endeavouring to encourage self-direction?	✓
Have I limited my assessment to a 'medical' explanatory model alone?	✗
Do the processes that I use privilege my understanding alone (for example, documentation, reviews, assessments, care planning)?	✗
Have the processes I utilised meant that the person I am working with knows the same information as I do?	✓
Have I enquired as to what the person has discovered about what works and what does not work for them?	✓
Does the intervention or support I provide support a learning environment for the client?	✓
Because of the support I offer, can I articulate what I am learning from the client?	✓
Connectedness – Disconnectedness	
Does the environment of support that I/we provide require a person to participate through their illness identity?	✗
Does the support or environment that I/we create help someone to connect with their citizenship (with same roles, expectations, responsibilities/rights and opportunities as everyone else)?	✓
Does the support or intervention provided reinforce a sense of being a recipient of services alone?	✗
Does the support or intervention help connect a person with a sense of contribution to other relationships and/or community?	✓
Is there a dominance of illness-saturated environments within the support structures that I provide (for example, drop-in centres, groups, centre based-support)?	✗
Have I considered how other people without a mental illness/support service would access the community before I create a 'service' response?	✓
Have I enquired as to 'what gets in the way' for a person to access the community before providing access through a mental health service response?	✓
Does the support I offer connect a person to relationships that are not paid?	✓
Does the support or intervention that I/we provide potentially connect a person to relationships beyond those who experience a mental illness?	✓

References

Australian Government (2010). 'Mental Health and Wellbeing – Policies', http://www.health.gov.au/internet/mentalhealth/publishing.nsf/Content/policies-lp-1, date accessed 8 November 2011.

Barrett, R. J. (1998). 'The Schizophrenic and the Liminal Persona in Modern Society', *Culture, Medicine and Psychiatry*, XXII, 465–94.

Calaprice, A. (2005). *The New Quotable Einstein* (Princeton, New Jersey: Princeton University Press).

Davidson, L. (2003). *Living Outside Mental Illness: Qualitative Studies of Recovery in Schizophrenia* (New York: New York University Press).

Deegan, P. (1988). 'Recovery: The Lived Experience of Rehabilitation', *Psychosocial Rehabilitation Journal*, 11(4), 11–19.

Estroff, S. E. (1993). 'Identity, Disability, and Schizophrenia: The Problem of Chronicity', in S. Lindenbaum and M. Lock (eds), *Knowledge, Power, and Practice: The Anthropology of Medicine and Everyday Life* (Berkeley & Los Angeles: University of California Press), 247–86.

European Union (2010). 'Health-EU. The Public Health Portal of the European Union, http://ec.europa.eu/health-eu/health_problems/mental_health, date accessed 26 November 2010.

Glover, H. (2007). 'Lived Experience Perspectives', in R. King, C. Lloyd and T. Meehan (eds), *Handbook of Psychosocial Rehabilitation* (Oxford: Blakwell Publishing).

Glover, H. (2009). *Unpacking Practices that Support People in their Efforts of Recovery, Level One Workbook* (Brisbane: Enlightened Consultants).

C. A. Griffiths and P. Ryan (2008). 'Recovery and Lifelong Learning: Interrelated Processes', *The International Journal of Psychosocial Rehabilitation*, XIII(1), 51–6.

Harding, C., Brooks, G., Ashikaga, T., Strauss, J. and Breier, A. (1987). 'The Vermont Longitudinal Study of Persons with Severe Mental Illness. I: Methodology, Study, Sample and Overall Status 32 Years Later', *American Journal of Psychiatry*, CIV (6), 727–35.

University of Hertfordshire and Hertfordshire Partnership Foundation NHS Trust (2008). *Recovery: Four Individual Experiences* (Hemel Hempstead: Serious Media Ltd.).

Jeffs, S. (2010). *Flying with Paper Wings* (North Carlton, Victoria: The Vulgar Press).

Johnstone, L. (2000). *Users and Abusers of Psychiatry* (London, UK: Routledge).

Kuhn, T. (1962). *The Structure of Scientifc Revolution* (Chicago: University of Chicago Press).

Mental Health Commission (2009). http://www.mhc.govt.nz, date accessed 26 November 2010.

Myers, N. L. (2010). 'Culture, Stress and Recovery from Schizophrenia: Lessons from the Field for Global Mental Health', *Cult Med Psychiatry*, XXXIV, 500–28.

Onken, S., Dumont, J., Ridgway, P. and Dornan, D. (2002). *Mental Health Recovery: What Heklps and What Hinders?* (New York: NASMHPD Office of Technical Assistance S. R. Network).

Roberts, G. (2007). 'Recovery: Our Common Purpose', *Advances in Psychiatric Treatment*, XIII, 397–99.

SAMHSA (2010). 'Substance Abuse and Mental Health Administration', http://www.samhsa.gov (home page), date accessed 26 November 2010.

Sartorius, N. (2002) 'Iatrogenic Stigma of Mental Illness', *British Medical Journal*, CCCXXIV (7532), 1470–1.

Scottish Recovery network (2009). 'Journeys of Recovery: Stories of Hope and Recovery from Long-Term Mental Health Problems', http://www.scottishrecovery.net, date accessed 8 November 2011.

Sullivan, W. (1994). 'A Long and Winding Road: The Process of Recovery from Severe Mental Illness', *Innovations and Research*, III(3), 19–27.

Summerfield, D. (2001). 'Does Psychiatry Stigmatise?', *J R Soc Med*, XCIV, 148–9.

Taylor, E. W. (2008). 'Transformative Learning Theory', *New Directions for Adult and Continuing Education*, 119, 5–15.

Tooth, B., Kalyanasundarm, V. and Glover, H. (2003). 'Factors Consumers Identify as Important to Recovery from Schizophrenia', *Australasian Psychiatry*, XI, 70–7.

Topor, A. (2001). *Managing the Contradication-Recovery from Severe Mental Disorders*, N. B. Language Makers, Trans. (Stockholm: Stockholm University, Department of Social Work).

Tsao, C., Tummala, A. and Roberts, L. (2008). 'Stigma in Mental Health Care', *Academic Psychiatry*, XXXII, 70–2.

World Health Organisation (2011). 'Mental Health: A State of Well-Being', http://www.who.int/features/factfiles/mental_health/en/index.html, date accessed 2 December 2011.

Zucconi, A. (2008). 'From Illness to Health, Well-Being and Empowerment: The Person-Centered Paradigm Shift from Patient to Client', in B. Levitt (ed.), *Reflections on Human Potential: Bridging the Person-Centred Approach and Positive Psychology* (PCCS Books, Ross on Wye: Hertfordshire, UK).

2

TREE: Towards Recovery, Empowerment and Experiential Expertise of Users of Psychiatric Services

Wilma Boevink

The burgeoning user moment in the Netherlands

The user movement in psychiatry has a lot to offer, more than we have been aware of so far. In the Netherlands, we take initiatives to strengthen our position and offer a different perspective on living with severe human distress with long-term mental illness or psychiatric disorders. We develop training courses for professionals in psychiatry. We start self-help groups and educate and train fellow users of psychiatry who want to integrate their experiences in professional roles. User-initiated projects are gaining in popularity and in substance. In countless areas, we have created activities on our own initiative. The underlying motivation is the conviction that our personal and collective experiences will lead to new insights regarding severe mental suffering and care (Boevink and Escher 2001, Boevink 2007, Boevink and Corstens 2011, Coleman 1999, Lehmann 2004). We are confident that we can contribute to building psychiatric services that are more supportive and human than the existing one's. Self-help and user initiatives in psychiatry are a response to the fact that our individuality, our experience and our knowledge are not yet adequately represented within mainstream psychiatry. For us, the emphasis is increasingly being placed on self-determination, our own responsibility and personal efforts, rather than devoting our strength to railing against the power of other stakeholders and their agendas.

Until now, there has been no general overview of European user and survivor initiatives unlike in the USA with the Consumer-Operated Services Program Multisite Research Initiative (COSP 2004). There is no account of the strategies we use, the experiences gained have yet to be collated and no solid scientific basis for our methods has been established. To contribute to the development of knowledge in the area of initiatives of users of psychiatry, long-term mental healthcare users in the Netherlands developed TREE – *'Towards Recovery, Empowerment and experiential Expertise'* – by, for and with persons with long-term and severe mental health problems.

Recovery

Persons labelled 'chronically mentally ill' can and do recover, whatever the general, negative, idea about them might be (Anthony 1993, Boevink, Plooy and van Rooijen 2006a, Deegan 1993). Recovery refers to the personal process of persons living with mental vulnerabilities in which they try to give new sense and meaning to their lives beyond the devastating effects of mental suffering. The recovery concept puts an end to the idea that you have to be 'cured' and without psychiatric symptoms to (be allowed to) participate in society. Whether prostheses ('mental wheelchairs') are needed or not, it is perfectly possible for people with psychiatric disabilities to occupy significant and valued roles in society. Recovery is about giving meaning to whatever it is you are overwhelmed with and about no longer letting the symptoms control your entire life. To recover means, on the one hand, not accepting the label of being 'untreatable' or 'therapy resistant' and, on the other hand, not or no longer fooling yourself that everything is all right in your life. Recovery means having the courage to face what is going on in your life and to accept there is extra and hard work to do. And of course it means actually starting working. To get to know your talents and possibilities, but also your vulnerabilities and less positive sides. To dare to have hope again and to (also) look towards the future. To dare to rely on your own strength and in your own way.

Empowerment

Recovery and empowerment are closely related. Recovery is not possible without empowerment and it is at the same time an empowering process. Empowerment is the development of the ability of people to wrestle their way out of hopeless situations and find new ways in life. In doing so, they learn by themselves how to choose ways of coping with new challenges and the kind of support they want.

Experiential expertise

To gain confidence with your own strengths and then develop and expand them, one needs experiential knowledge: knowledge about what helps and hinders in one's own recovery process. In our opinion, recovery and empowerment lean on experiential knowledge and expertise. People with the experience of severe and long-term human distress all have their own unique story. This story includes the meaning they give to their problems and the strategies developed to handle these problems. This is the so-called personal experiential knowledge. All these individual stories together form collective experiential knowledge: knowledge about how it is to live with mental vulnerability and its consequences. If one is capable of passing on this knowledge to others in any form, then we use the word experiential expertise. Experiential expertise is essential for the recovery of persons labelled mentally ill. On an individual level, it helps empower fellow sufferers in their quest for their own strength(s). On a higher level, it paves the way for user influence in improving mental healthcare services. TREE is a company developed and run by experiential experts. Participants in TREE activities have the opportunity to develop their own skills as experiential experts.

The TREE programme

TREE brings together the strategies and methods users and survivors of psychiatry have developed and which are thought to account for their success. It aims at enabling people with psychiatric disabilities to support each other towards recovery, empowerment and experiential expertise, thus enhancing their ability to manage their own lives and to counter their marginalisation in society (Boevink et al. 2002, Boevink 2006b). To this end, the programme enables its participants to exchange experiences and offer mutual support. It also encourages them to develop knowledge and to use such knowledge by making it available to others. The programme promotes user/survivor-led change within mental healthcare organisations towards recovery-based services. Finally, TREE has an important destigmatising influence: research shows that the most effective way of combating stigma is to bring the general public in direct contact with the stigmatized group ('to know one is to tolerate one') (Corrigan ct al. 2001). TREE participants are trained to make and tell their stories to a range of target groups, among them subgroups from the general public. In the TREE programme, participants develop, transform and disseminate experiential knowledge. They perform these tasks themselves, as volunteers or in paid jobs in the mental healthcare organisations where the programme is implemented. If necessary, they hire others, for example, mental healthcare professionals, as prostheses to enable them to perform their tasks.

TREE may sound self-evident, but it becomes very special if one takes into account the fact that the programme is for, by and with persons with long-term mental health problems, such as psychiatric disabilities. They often struggle with multiple and complex problems in several domains of life and most of them have impressive patient careers in psychiatry. As a consequence, they face dependency, lack of self-confidence and self-esteem, loss of control over their lives, loss of meaningful identity and greater social vulnerability.

There are no other criteria to enter the programme than to have (the courage to have) some interest in what the programme is about. We do not know which factors predict success. Perhaps it is better not to know. The programme is developed in order to create opportunities for recovery and empowerment and to facilitate whoever wants to make use of these opportunities. Inherent to this goal is that everybody can participate. Practice will show for whom it is a successful opportunity and for whom it is not. The programme is open to all users and survivors of long-term mental healthcare. There are no inclusion criteria, no demands, no examination and it can be used as often and as long (or as short) as one likes.

Stories in TREE

A person with a psychiatric disability can take part as a member of a self-help group, as a student of one of the courses, a volunteer or as a paid experiential expert. The programme offers the opportunity to

- communicate with others about experiences that are overwhelming;
- create some distance from these experiences and reflect upon them (develop one's own narrative);
- make a we-story out of several I-stories (experiential story);
- make the experiential narrative useful for disseminating knowledge to fellow users and survivors of psychiatry, mental healthcare professionals and others; and
- participate as a (paid) trainer or lecturer in training programmes.

The underlying principle is that an important element in recovering from long-term mental illness is to develop and pass on narratives (Baart 2002, Boevink 2006c, Chamberlin 1979). To make and to tell a narrative enables us to overcome whatever it is we are overwhelmed with, for instance a psychosis, because it empowers us to recover our sense of self (Herman 1992). Through telling our story, we grow from being a disorder to becoming a person trying to deal with life (Boevink 2006d, Ridgeway 2002). And it enables us to learn to formulate what it is we need to recover (from). To develop your own narrative and compare it with the narratives of other users and survivors of psychiatry is the beginning of building experiential knowledge. A collective story develops out of several individual narratives. To this end, we look for underlying principles, for what we have in common and for what distinguishes us from one another. Finally, the experiential story is transformed and used for knowledge dissemination in training programmes and courses.

Basically the programme consists of

- self-help groups and working groups;
- training, courses and workshops for fellow users and survivors of psychiatry;
- training programmes for professional caregivers;
- training for professionals and users together; and
- consulting and coaching of TREE innovations in organisations in mental healthcare.

The TREE team

The TREE team consists of 60 persons from all over the country in different phases of their recovery process and in different phases of their development as experiential experts. An important condition for joining the team is to have had a psychiatric (serious, long-term and disrupting daily life) past and present. TREE has experienced members, veterans and trainees. Responsibility for the implementation of an entire TREE programme in a mental healthcare setting lies with the veterans in cooperation with the TREE coordinator.

Participants play different roles: there are people who support a recovery group, participants who present their recovery story and, for example, team members who take overall responsibility for providing a training course or seminar. Of course, combinations of tasks are possible. One can still be a trainee concerned with one competency, but at the same time be working relatively autonomously on another task. For instance: a member can have shared responsibility with a co-facilitator of a self-help group (there are always two facilitators for each group), but still be under tight supervision as a lecturer about recovery. The TREE team has a system of coaching in inter/supervision. Veterans support juniors, and mutual support among all is stimulated strongly. Not just in the recovery self-help groups, but also within the TREE team, mutual support and self-help is a powerful source of resilience.

TREE is unusual in that there is no traditional distinction between 'professionals' who do the work and 'patients' who are helped or 'served'. It is the psychiatric services users themselves who are the actors and who, if they want to, develop into the one's who carry out work in paid jobs. Most TREE members started by working on their own recovery in a recovery self-help group and then, at one point, chose to further develop their knowledge and skills as TREE members. Several members are now working in paid jobs in psychiatric institutions or other organisations as experiential experts. We always strive to do these jobs while still staying a member of TREE, thus guaranteeing ongoing learning and exchange of experiences and support. This ongoing contact (and contract) has the advantage that the members are dispatched for temporary jobs to other organisations than their own or even other countries. This keeps them alert and inspired and also prevents narrow-mindedness and a feeling of powerlessness when pioneering within one's own organisation.

Informing fellow users

Usually, the first phase of TREE interventions in psychiatric institutions consists of visiting its patients and telling them our own stories, thus allowing them to familiarise themselves with the hopeful perspective of recovery. We visit people in places with which they are familiar and where they feel comfortable. We try to fit the information sessions into their daily routine and we adapt our ways of communicating to each different audience. We try to ensure that the people providing the information share experiences with their audience. Providing information to people living in a sheltered housing facility, for example, is ideally carried out by people who also live or have lived in such a facility. The information meetings are, of course, not obligatory. All that the facilitators can do is to create the opportunity for the audience to become curious or to be tempted (to open up) by something new. That in itself is often a big task for people who have ground to a hopeless halt after years of loss and suffering.

Kick-off meeting

After contacting the people living in the psychiatric institution, a kick-off meeting is organised. These meetings are chaired by a TREE team consisting of a senior trainer, a trainee who presents the experiential story and two participants in TREE projects elsewhere. We invite a maximum of 25 users, family members, carers, managers and policy-makers to the meeting. Users must always make up at least half plus one of those present at the meeting to ensure that they are properly represented and that their voice is heard. In order to make it possible for people to attend, it is made clear that one can leave the meeting for a break and come back whenever one wants. It is pointed out that people's limitations in terms of energy or concentration, for example, should be taken seriously, that the TREE team is familiar with them and knows how important it is to respect them. The purpose of the meeting is to present a clear explanation of TREE so as to lay the basis for local TREE projects and activities.

The meeting often takes up a whole morning (or an afternoon or an evening) and is divided into three parts:

• In the first part, the meaning of the three concepts (recovery, empowerment and experiential expertise) is explained in a brief information session using experiential stories. After the experiential stories, the senior trainer asks those present to think of an over-whelming experience in their own lives from which they have had to recover. He or she then asks each person which strategies they used to bring about that recovery and, above all, which strategies helped and which did not. The responses are then collected and written on a flip chart; the aim is to show that there is (virtually) no difference between the strategies used by people with and without psychiatric disabilities.
• The second part is devoted to TREE activities elsewhere in the coun-try. These are described briefly and specifically, so that those present are able to form a picture of them. A number of participants from other locations are also interviewed about their participation in the TREE activities in their own region.
• In the third part, a basis is laid for TREE within the host institution. Those present are then invited to make known their own preferences and wishes in smaller groups. Based on the outcome, the TREE team then writes a project proposal.

The kick-off meeting is often also the place where people register for the proposed activity. Contacts are also established at these meetings with enthusiastic professionals who can play the role of ambassadors later on in the project.

The recovery self-help group: developing strengths

This group forms the basis for the programme. It consists of a maximum of eight participants plus two experiential experts to act as facilitators. They meet for two hours every two weeks. The workshop activities are based on recovery and empowerment. The emphasis in the discussion of personal experiences is not on problems and illness, but on strengths and possibilities. This is not to say that mental suffering is denied or ignored; the group develops ways of increasing each member's strengths and possibilities so they are better able to deal with their suffering. It is not a therapy group, but a self-help group.

During the meetings, which have a set structure, participants are given the opportunity to talk about their daily lives. This enables them to learn to talk about their experiences using self-chosen words and to learn to listen to each other. Both are skills that seem rarely to be used and often forgotten when living as a chronic patient in a psychiatric institution. The participants share experiences and give each other support and advice. In this way, they experience the positive value of their own experiences and learn to see them as a source of knowledge. The different contributions and discussions are recorded in the minutes of the meeting. This is an important part of the meetings: discussing the meetings helps people to look at their own experiences from a distance and to place them in a broader context. In this way, themes can be identified on the basis of everyday personal experiences. These themes are then discussed in more depth at subsequent meetings.

The next step is to make individual experiential stories based on the answers to questions such as, 'Who am I? What is it that I have to learn to live with? How can I help myself? How can others help me?' For this purpose, the participants prepare a presentation for fellow users outside the group. The idea is that they tell the audience about their own recovery experiences and explain what recovery from mental illness can mean. The fact that there is now an audience of relative outsiders means their experiences have to be moulded into a coherent and accessible story, with a beginning and an end.

The reports of the discussions in the group can also be used to enable people to mix their own experiences with those of others. This integration of personal stories into one collective story is not the same thing as aiming for consensus. On the contrary, the whole point of experiential knowledge is that it describes different standpoints, overlaps and differences. Experiential knowledge should not reduce these complexities, but make them understandable. Finally, participants are offered training in constructing stories and presentation techniques to help them convey recovery stories to other people. The recovery self-help groups are the basis for the implementation of recovery-oriented programmes in psychiatric institutions. They form a potential source for new experiential experts who, later in the process, can become the new leaders of the innovative changes in their own institution.

The recovery seminar

One of the ways of transferring experiential knowledge is by organising seminars on recovery. The seminar programme targets patients receiving long-term care and their professional mental healthcare workers. They can only take part if they come as a pair (patient and professional). The aim is to familiarise participants with the meaning of recovery and to teach them to apply that meaning in their own lives. All the trainers are experiential experts based on their career as users of long-term care.

During the introductory session, participants are interviewed about their lives, their experiences, their dreams and their frustrations. The trainers focus on what patients and professionals have in common, with a view to blurring the traditional dividing line between the two groups. During the morning, there is also information transfer about recovery, including through the use of experiential stories. In the ensuing discussion, the aim is to generate a conversation between the patients. This is usually the first time in their lives that they hear about hopeful recovery experiences from fellow patients, and they often are very eager to talk about them. The professional workers are (respectfully and implicitly) placed in the position of audience. They are given the chance to witness the sometimes enormously positive changes that patients undergo when they first come into contact with recovery and with experiential experts.

In the afternoon, based on an experiential story, the focus is on the relationship between patient and professional and the development of the recovery concept. The participants can then practise more personal interaction with their pairs; based on the idea that recovery support is a two-way process, the members of each pair are invited to talk to each other. Both write down a positive and a less positive experience they have had with the other person and then read it out loud. It is difficult for patients to mention a less positive experience concerning the professional, because they are generally not accustomed to this or do not have the courage to give feedback about such an experience to their professional carer. For professional workers in psychiatry, it is often extremely difficult to produce a non-therapeutic comment, one with a more personal input; they are not used to it as they have learnt to maintain a professional distance in their contact with clients.

'Making a start on recovery' course

'Making a start on recovery' is a familiarisation course on the meaning of the concept of 'recovery' for patients using long-term psychiatric care. Recovery is to do with learning to live with persistent (vulnerability to) mental health problems. The course is intended to serve as an initial familiarisation with the concepts of recovery and rehabilitation, to help people gain experience in discussing these concepts and to prompt people into an awareness of their own recovery process. The course does not involve any homework or reading work: the entire course consists of a structured discussion with other participants and with the experiential experts who are the course leaders. The course consists of five meetings: each lasting two hours, spread over a maximum of ten weeks. Each meeting has the same structure: introduction; presentation by guest lecturer; questions; exercises; close. The five meetings are based around the themes of the meaning of recovery; support with recovery; traps; the role of professionals in recovery; and how to continue your own recovery process.

These themes are also the themes of the first series of meetings of the recovery self-help group. This means that a participant can easily become a guest lecturer on the 'Making a start on recovery' course. This enables them to practise in different roles and to experience how life as a psychiatric patient can also mean having rich sources of knowledge to use. The guest lecturers are interviewed and supported in preparing for their task. They receive payment for their visit in the course so as to not interfere with whatever income they have. Participation in the course is free of charge. There is place for five to seven participants.

The 'Recovery-Supportive Care' training programme

A basic course, 'Recovery and Recovery-Supportive Care', was developed jointly by experiential experts and rehabilitation trainers. It was developed for professionals for whom the terms 'recovery' and 'recovery-supportive care' are relatively new. The course lasts for two days.

On Day 1, the TREE concepts are presented, with the aim of helping participants to

1. learn about the concepts of recovery, empowerment and experiential expertise;
2. gain an insight into the meaning of these concepts in their own lives so that they can imagine how those concepts might take form in the lives of their patients.

The programme on Day 1 consists of teaching the TREE concepts, both theoretically and through an experiential story. The day is also focused on familiarisation with the meaning of recovery in the lives of course participants. A number of exercises and assignments are carried out in small groups.

On Day 2, the meaning of recovery-supportive care is added to the personal meaning of recovery, with the aim of giving participants

1. knowledge of what recovery-supportive care is and developing a number of ideas about what it can mean in their day-to-day work;
2. knowledge of the relationship between recovery-supportive care, treatment and rehabilitation, and exchanging first ideas about how treatment and support can be changed through the use of recovery-supportive care.

The programme on Day 2 begins with the homework assignment from Day 1. The concept of recovery-supportive care is explained and discussed. Recovery-supportive care, rehabilitation and treatment and their mutual relationships are then explored through knowledge transfer, experiential stories and exercises.

Day 1 is led entirely by experiential experts from the TREE team. On Day 2, the training team consists of an experiential expert and a rehabilitation trainer. The course can be given to a maximum of 14 people. This might be an existing team from a mental healthcare organisation, or a mixed group with professionals from different parts of the organisation. Each day goes from 10 am to 5 pm.

Towards evidence for our wisdom

In the Netherlands, the TREE programme, or parts of it, has become increasingly popular among people with psychiatric disabilities themselves as well as among care providers. Most mental healthcare organisations have started to support their users to implement the programme. A nation-wide operating team of experiential experts is now frequently hired to provide kick-off meetings, support users and survivors in their recovery and in building recovery narratives, coach persons with psychiatric disabilities to become experiential experts, train fellow users and survivors of psychiatry and professionals, give lectures and design new programme modules. From 2004 to 2007, a randomised, controlled trial of TREE (n = 81) versus care (struggling) as usual (n = 82) in patients with severe mental illness was conducted at four Dutch sites. Follow-up measures were collected at 24 months. Primary patient outcome measures were empowerment, mental health confidence, loneliness and quality of life. Secondary patient outcomes were self-reported symptoms and care needs. The primary process outcome was successful implementation and sustainability (continued engagement more than 50 per cent of the programme over the two-year period).

The programme was implemented successfully and sustained over the course of 24 months in the majority of participants. Despite the limited number of participants, the experimental condition was associated with small positive impacts on mental health confidence and self-reported symptoms and no negative impacts. User-developed/run recovery programmes can be implemented in a sustainable fashion alongside traditional mental healthcare services; they are furthermore open to evaluation by traditional trial methodologies. Results suggest that they may aid recovery processes.

TREE for the future

The development of new training and courses continues. The themes for training are numerous and there is great need for TREE in psychiatry, both for users and for professionals. A number of courses have been developed since the early years with regard to making and telling stories, coping with voices and growing beyond self-harm. TREE also experiments with new formats, like theatre, photography and voice exercises. At the same time, training experiential experts has developed further. The training consists of on-the-job competency education and training under supervision of senior TREE members. Finally, TREE grows in its knowledge and use of the possibilities of vocational rehabilitation, especially when it comes to creating spaces for slower rehabilitation processes and being paid for first attempts without losing the safety of one's social pension.

In TREE, we develop experiential knowledge. We pass that knowledge on to others: to the next generation of care service users, to give them strength and hope; to professionals in mental healthcare, to learn to hear our voices; to people outside mental healthcare altogether, so that our human face be seen.

The TREE programme is facilitated by theTrimbos Institute (www.trimbos. org) and the Rehabilitation '92 Foundation, an organisation aiming to introduce and implement the psychiatric rehabilitation approach of the Centre for Psychiatric Rehabilitation of Boston University in the Dutch Mental Health Care System. Research on recovery and empowerment received financial support from the Foundation for Mental Health in Utrecht. The TREE effectiveness study was made possible by the Netherlands Organization for Health Research and Development (www.ZONMw.nl/en) and by the Foundation for Sheltered Housing Accommodation in Utrecht (SBWU).

References

Anthony, W. A. (1993). 'Recovery from Mental Illness: The Guiding Vision of the Mental Health Service System in the 1990s', *Psychosocial Rehabilitation Journal*, XVI, 4, 11–23.

Baart, I. (2002). *Ziekte en zingeving. Een onderzoek naar chronische ziekte en subjectiviteit [The Shaping of Identity in Illness. A Study on Chronic Illness and Subjectivity]* (Assen: Van Gorcum).

Boevink, W. and Escher, S. (2001). *Making Self-Harm Understandable* (Bemelen: Stichting Positieve Gezondheidszorg/Foundation for Positive Health Care).

Boevink, W., van Beuzekom, J., Gaal, E., Jadby, A., Jong, F., Klein Bramel, M., Kole, M., te Loo, N., Scholtus, S. and van der Wal, C. (2002). *Samen werken aan herstel. Van ervaringen delen naar kennis overdragen* [Working Together on Recovery: from Sharing Experiences to Implementing Knowledge] (Utrecht: Trimbos-Institute).

Boevink, W., Plooy, A. and van Rooijen, S (2006a). *Herstel, Empowerment en Ervaringsdeskundigheid van mensen met psychische aandoeningen* [Recovery, Empowerment and Experiential Expertise of Persons with Mental Health Problems] (Amsterdam: SWP).

Boevink, W. (2006b). *Stories of Recovery. Working together towards Experiential Knowledge in Mental Health Care*. (Utrecht: Trimbos-institute).

Boevink, W. (2006c). 'From Alien to Actor'. Lecture Held During the Public Hearing on The Green Paper on Mental Health, European Parliament, Brussels, June 8, and ENUSP web site: www.enusp.org/documents/boevink_alien.pdf, date accessed 14 June 2011.

Boevink, W. (2006d). 'From Being a Disorder to Dealing with Life. An Experiential Exploration of the Association between Trauma and Psychosis', *Schizophrenia Bulletin*, XXXII, 1, 17–19.

Boevink, W. (2007). 'Survival, the Art of Living and Knowledge to Pass on. Recovery, Empowerment and experiential Expertise of Persons with Severe Mental Health Problems', in P. Stastny and P. Lehmann (eds), *Alternatives beyond Psychiatry* (Berlin: Peter Lehmann Publishing).

Boevink, W. and Corstens, D. (2011). 'My Body Remembers; I Refused. Childhood Trauma, Dissocation and Psychosis', in J. Geekie, R. Randal, D. Lampshire and J. Read (eds), *Experiencing Psychosis* (London: Routledge).

Chamberlin, J. (1979). *On Our Own: Patient-Controlled Alternatives to the Mental Health System* (New York: McGraw-Hill).

Coleman, R. (1999). *Recovery: An Alien Concept* (Gloucester, UK: Handsell Publishing).

Consumer-Operated Services Program Multisite Research Initiative (COSP) (2004). http://www.mimh.edu/cstprogramarchive/consumer%20op/, date accessed 14 December 2011.

Corrigan, P. W., River, L. P., Lundin, R. K., Penn, D. L., Uphoff-Wasowski, K., Campion, J., Mathisen, J., Cagnon, C., Bergman, M., Goldstein, H. and Kubiak, M. A. (2001). 'Three Strategies for Changing Attributions about Severe Mental Illness', *Schizophrenia Bulletin*, XXVII, 2, 187–95.

Deegan, P. E. (1993). 'Recovering our Sense of Value after Being Labeled Mentally Ill', *Journal of Psychosocial Nursing*, XXXI, 4, 7–11.

Herman, J. (1992). *Trauma and Recovery. The Aftermath of Violence – from Domestic Abuse to Political Terror* (New York: Basic Books).

Lehmann, P. (2004). *Coming Off Psychiatric Drugs. Successful Withdrawal from Neuroleptics, Antidepressants, Lithium, Carbamazepine and Tranquilizers* (Berlin: Peter Lehmann Publishing).

Ridgeway, P. (2002). 'Restoring Psychiatric Disability: Learning from First Person Recovery Narratives', *Psychiatric Rehabilitation Journal*, XXIV, 335–43.

3
Wellness Recovery Action Planning (WRAP)

Barbara Evans and Kate Sault

Wellness Recovery Action Planning (WRAP) is a self-management tool developed in the USA by Mary Ellen Copeland and based on the principles of recovery. Our WRAP journey in Hampshire started in 2003 when Mary Ellen Copeland came to England to facilitate a five-day WRAP training programme for a group made up half of mental health professionals and half of people who use mental health services. The training was both challenging and inspiring. The work of WRAP is firmly embedded in the context of recovery, a philosophy of care that has evolved over the past ten years through the international voice of service users. WRAP can be defined as a tool that can aid an individual's recovery and its underpinning principles support the recovery approach. WRAP is a systematic way of monitoring wellness, times of being less well and times when experiences are uncomfortable and distressing. It also includes details of how an individual would like others to support them at these different times.

After this initial training, we established a steering group composed of a mix of professionals and service users. At the start, there were two or three services users. Now services users, employed by various organisations throughout Hampshire and attached to the project as WRAP Ambassadors, make up more that 50 per cent of the group. The steering group meets approximately every six weeks and all major decisions are ratified by the group before implementation. The WRAP mission statement, developed by the steering group, is: to develop a new type of worker who will train and equip both staff and people who use mental health services to facilitate the universal availability of WRAP as a self-management tool within all areas of the Southern Health Foundation Trust.

The development of WRAP has been achieved primarily through the coordination and delivery of awareness raising and WRAP training. The aim has been to equip staff and service users with the skills they need to introduce and support service users in the development of their own WRAP. Staff and people with lived experience are trained together as WRAP facilitators. This has been identified as a way of learning and understanding WRAP that breaks down some of the stigma related to the 'them and us' culture often generated in patient/professional relationships. It has also increased recognition that we all fall on the continuum of mental well-being which can hugely impact the effectiveness of our work and home lives.

The WRAP approach is strongly linked to national mental health policy in the UK. In 2007, the *Mental Health Policy Implementation Guide* (DOH 2007) recommended that all who staff, whether in health or social care, should learn about and adopt Ten Essential Shared Capabilities and the Recovery approach, including WRAP. In his introduction to the new national strategy 'No Health without Mental Health', Andrew Lansley states that 'Putting people who use services at the heart of everything we do – "No decision about me without me" – is the governing principle. Care should be personalized to reflect people's needs, not those of the professional or the system' (DOH 2011, p. 3). WRAP supports this objective in its entirety. Similarly, WRAP is a tool that can 'help clinicians to engage people in decisions about personalizing their treatment and to respect their wishes as far as possible, not least because this can make a real difference to outcomes' (DOH 2011, p. 32).

WRAP is based on Copeland's five key principles of recovery (Copeland 1997):

1. Hope: people who experience health difficulties get as well as they can, stay well and go on to meet their life dreams and goals.
2. Personal Responsibility: it is up to you, with the assistance of others, to take action and do what needs to be done to keep yourself well.
3. Education: learning all you can about what you are experiencing so you can make good decisions about all aspects of your life.
4. Self-advocacy: effectively reaching out to others so that you can get what it is that you need, want and deserve to support your wellness and recovery.
5. Support: while working towards your wellness is up to you, receiving support from others, and giving support to others, will help you feel better and enhance the quality of your life.

Lived experience of mental ill-health and/or other-long term conditions is core to the philosophy of WRAP and runs through all areas of our work. An essential criterion for the role of 'WRAP project support' within the team is that post holders have experience of using mental health services. Service users are members of the project steering group. All training is co-facilitated by a service user. Service users who have undertaken WRAP training support others in developing their WRAPs individually and in groups. They regularly co-present WRAP at conferences and workshops, and are involved in research in relation to WRAP. Work placements within the project for service users include administrative support and help with general team developments.

A key feature of WRAP is that it is developed and owned by the individual and not the organisation responsible for support or treatment. The individual is placed firmly in the driver's seat rather than 'locked in the boot' (Glover 2002). WRAP is about emphasising holistic health, wellness, strengths, interests, abilities and social support. It focuses on the individual's strengths and builds on them as well as encourages personal responsibility and self-management, resulting in individuals having more control over their lives. It is also a way of helping people to build support structures, make contingency plans and action plan.

WRAP training asks all participants, including staff, to develop their own WRAP, as we acknowledge that we all have a responsibility for our wellness. By doing this, we feel that staff, having experienced the process themselves, are better equipped to promote WRAP to service users. This exploratory style of training is relatively new within our service and many staff (and teams) have reported the benefits of having their own WRAP and this style of training. The interface between staff and service users has changed as a result of the training, empowering individuals, enhancing the therapeutic relationship and raising self-awareness in relation to the steps both staff and service users need to adopt to stay well.

The WRAP programme which has been developed in Hampshire is made up of eight sections. The individual works through each section at their own pace, starting with any section depending on their preference. However it is suggested to focus on section 1 (Wellness) first.

The eight WRAP sections

1. **Wellness**: this is where you explore what wellness means to you and what you are like when you are at your very best. It helps you not to lose sight of who you can be.
2. **Wellness toolbox**: This is where you identify the things that can help you maintain your optimum level of wellness.

3. **Daily maintenance plan**: This is where you think about the things you need to do on a regular basis to maximise your wellness.
4. **Triggers**: These are external events or circumstances that may undermine your well-being. You identify and list your personal triggers and develop an action plan for dealing with them.
5. **Early warning signs**: These are subtle signs of emotional and behavioural change that indicate to you or others that you are becoming less well. You identify and list your early warning signs and develop an action plan for dealing with them.
6. **When things are breaking down**: These can be feelings, behaviours and physical signs that indicate to you that things are more serious. You or someone else may need to take immediate action to prevent things from worsening.
7. **A crisis plan**: This is a comprehensive plan that is written when you are well. It includes information for others about the kind of help you would like if you feel less able to cope with life.
8. **A post-crisis plan**: This section offers an opportunity to review how the crisis plan worked and focuses on what steps you may want to take following a period of crisis or when you have been unable to cope with life. It looks at what changes need to be made, what can be learnt and what will help you to maximise your well-being.

In the authors' experience, it is easier and a more positive experience to complete a WRAP when feeling well. It can be difficult if the person is not very well or in a crisis. A suggested way to start is to use an A4 ring-binder folder with eight file dividers, one for each of the WRAP sections. Participants are encouraged to be creative (for example, using photography, scrapbooking, arts and craft, digital story, video diary), to ask for ideas and comments from people that they trust or know well and to include previous work such as coping strategies, psychological work, care plan, goal setting or crisis planning. It is recommended to take your time, to think about each section carefully and review it regularly: a WRAP should be considered as work in progress. The key to the facilitation of WRAP is knowing the sections really well. Having done it personally is crucial, and means that you are not reliant on paperwork alone to later explain WRAP. The paperwork, which can be perceived as daunting, is merely there for explanation and inspiration rather than as a pathway that should be rigidly adhered to. Even when finished, changes can be made to the WRAP as individual circumstances change or simply if one changes one's mind. Indeed, the value of a WRAP plan is not just in the process of creating it, but in using it regularly, reviewing and developing it on the basis of further experience, so that it becomes a well-honed working tool. The plan for using WRAP is to put it into action at times of difficulty and amend it after significant life events, both positive and negative. These can then be more easily regarded as experiences to learn from – what worked, what did not, what we can do better for the future.

Train the trainer programme for sessional workers

The initial criterion for sessional workers' involvement is that they have a WRAP. The team then meets with the individual and works out a development plan including skills they have to offer, training that might be required and the type of involvement they would like to have. The team then offer a five-day 'Train the Trainer' programme, advertised as 'A fun and friendly environment in which you can learn to transform nervous fear into creative energy by understanding how groups work and learn, preparing and practicing presentation skills, finding what you are comfortable to share from your personal experiences'.

In addition to this training, on-the-job mentoring is offered, along with group and individual supervision. All service users working in the team are paid and fall within the Trust's work placement scheme which meets relevant Human Resources requirements.

> My role is to train people how to produce and use WRAP. I have one myself and it has helped me manage my health. I can include ways of dealing with my health that I have learnt from various treatments in the past. I can also include new ways to deal with new triggers that may appear in my life. WRAP is like a framework for my life, I use it to produce an action plan for my day. If I have a bad day, I can look in my WRAP and see what I am meant to be doing that day like washing and visiting friends.
>
> (A WRAP sessional worker)

Overcoming the barriers

WRAP is becoming increasingly embedded in the fabric of our local health system, with the recovery-focused approach having a significant effect on organisational culture.

> It removes some of the barriers between staff and service users reminding us that we all have needs, early warning signs, times of wellness and crisis.
>
> (A WRAP course delegate)

This has not however been achieved without overcoming a number of challenges along the way. Changing service culture in general has been a major issue. There is still a strong medical model of care within adult Mental Health Services in England. The power and control in the relationship between recipient and caregiver falls to the caregiver, with the medically qualified professional predominantly leading this. The WRAP teams have been working alongside colleagues to change this relationship to one of a more of an equal status where the giver of care takes more of a coaching role and the relationship is based on values of the recovery approach.

> I feel WRAP really helps to address the power balance between professionals and service users.
>
> (A WRAP course delegate)

Culture within a service is hard to shift and this takes time. WRAP has definitely been a vehicle that has helped this, primarily due to the fact that it is a tool the individual develops and owns. WRAP empowers an individual to explore themselves in depth, making it easier to articulate and share what helps and what does not in relation to their wellness at a given time. This means an individual is not relying on the caregiver for all the answers but becomes an expert in themselves.

> I think for some people it's an entirely new approach, and people that have been working in the services for 20 years or more ... might be familiar with some concepts of recovery, but this is such a comparatively new way of working ... that it might be a challenge for them ... to take it on board.
>
> (A WRAP course delegate)

There has been some confusion as to how WRAP fits within official policy recommendations on care planning recommendations, in England known as the Care Programme Approach (CPA). The CPA is the national framework for planning, assessing and reviewing an individual's care. We feel that WRAP does not and should not be appended to existing systems of care as it is not a service-driven tool but one owned by the individual. We recommend that elements of WRAP, if a service user chooses, be incorporated into a CPA to ensure that the individual's voice is heard. Also, if a CPA is of high quality, it should mirror aspects of WRAP.

Other common fears with the idea of service-user involvement include issues of confidentiality and boundaries stemming from the change in roles and responsibilities a service user has when becoming a WRAP co-facilitator. Time has been spent with teams discussing these issues and using areas where there is effective service-user involvement as examples of how it can and does work. Service-user involvement remains a key objective for the team and our aspiration is for WRAP led by service users in the near future.

An ongoing obstacle for some people has been the perceived amount of paperwork and number of sections in a WRAP. We have spent a lot of time developing our training to make it as creative as possible. We promote the fact that WRAP can be developed in numerous ways including pictorially, as a scrapbook, on a PC or hand-written – however the individual feels it would most usefully convey the information needed.

Evaluation: measuring outcomes

In our local services, clinical outcome measures associated with WRAP, such as the Mental Health Confidence Scale and the Empowerment Scale, are increasingly being used to identify the outcomes of individual interventions. The WRAP team is currently seeking a generic tool to be used across services but this is not an easy task as recovery is so personal and it is critical not to lose the essence of the individual's journey. A pilot study is currently underway to establish the benefits of the Recovery Star outcome measure. We have also been collating evidence using a DVD developed by service users for service users, regular newsletters consisting of service-user testimonies and digital storytelling to enable service users to illustrate their experiences of recovery and WRAP through self-created short films. Digital storytelling is a personal event or experience made into a short film. It is created by the storyteller who is taught new skills in order to tell their story. The storyteller uses still images, with or without words or a voice over, often with background music. These stories have been used personally by individuals, in training and at conferences. The power of an individual's story has been recognised by audiences as a far more effective way of illustrating recovery than a PowerPoint presentation.

Has WRAP made a difference?

In Hampshire, WRAP has had a substantial impact on enabling service users to feel empowered and more in control of their wellbeing. Some 500 staff members have been trained – from early intervention teams and in-patient services through to community mental health teams and rehabilitation services. The aim is to create a seamless model so that, wherever a person is in their journey through the service, they will have the support to develop and review their plan. To help achieve this, voluntary sector and service-user organisations are also able to access the training. An audit trail to describe the number of service users who have a WRAP was completed.

> To me, WRAP is very empowering – it is like having a mental thermostat and leads to better self-awareness too. I have been able to take control for the first time in my life.
>
> (A mental health service user)

> One of the greatest things that has resulted from creating my own personal WRAP is that I have greater understanding of myself. This understanding has made it possible for me to develop action plans which have helped me over and over again to maintain my wellness.
>
> (A mental health service user)

> I think part of it is to empower you yourself, to bring about your own mental state sort of thing. There are still things that I do that have helped me, and they're still the same as they were prior to doing the WRAP, but I think knowledge and introspection is power – power to affect your mental state.
>
> (A mental health service user)

As with any new initiative, challenges are to be expected. However these pale into insignificance when you speak to someone who has seen WRAP as 'life-changing'. Each year, we hold a Stakeholder Event which is an opportunity for stakeholders to network, hear from those with lived experience of WRAP and help plan future WRAP developments. The energy created from these events is amazing and something we are very proud of.

> Recovery means so many things to different people. Most people hear the word recovery and relate it to a broken leg in that it will get better. For me, recovery might never mean coming off medication or being symptom free, what it does mean for me includes looking at my life, finding ways to cope, knowing what is real, taking back responsibility and finally finding out who I am.
>
> (A mental health service user)

The authors would like to thank, for their contributions to this chapter, Sarah Richmond (Deputy WRAP Coordinator), Julia McKenzie (Project Support), the WRAP Co-facilitators and the WRAP Ambassadors, both service users and staff, in the HPFT.

References

Copeland, M. E. (1997). *Wellness Recovery Action Plan* (Dummerton, VT: Peach Press).
Department of Health (DOH) (2011). *No Health without Mental Health. A Cross-Government Mental Health Outcomes Strategy for People of All Ages*, Mental Health Division (Department of Health: London).
Department of Health (DOH) (2007). 'Mental Health Policy Implementation Guide: A Learning and Development Toolkit for the Whole of the Mental Health Workforce across Both Health and Social Care', http://www.dh.gov.uk/en/Publicationsandstatistics/Publications/PublicationsPolicyAndGuidance/DH_073682, date accessed 10 June 2011.
Glover, H. (2002). *A series of thoughts on Personal Recovery*. http://www.mhaca.org.au/2010resources/Personal%20recovery.pdf, date accessed 21 December 2011.

Further reading online

Mary Ellen Copeland's website *www.mentalhealthrecovery.com*, date accessed 14 June 2011.
The Scottish Recovery Network – WRAP pages http://www.scottishrecovery.net/WRAP/wellness-recovery-actions-planning.html, date accessed 14 June 2011.
Research project on self-managed care in which the Hampshire WRAP team participated: www.sdo.nihr.ac.uk/files/project/165-exec-summary.pdf, date accessed 14 June 2011.
The Joy of Appreciative Living http://appreciativeliving.com/, date accessed 14 June 2011.
The Recovery Star http://www.mhpf.org.uk/recoveryStar.asp, date accessed 14 June 2011.
The Digital Story Center, California www.storycenter.org, date accessed 14 June 2011.
Digital stories can be developed using free software, such as Photo Story 3. http://www.microsoft.com/windowsxp/using/digitalphotography/photostory/default.msp, date accessed 14 June 2011.

4

The Role of Mental Health Service Users in Recovery from Professional Stigma

Robert W. Surber

'I am a professional in recovery'. It is with this statement that I began a presentation I gave at a conference in 1996 to describe my efforts to employ mental health service users as direct service providers for the Citywide Case Management Team in San Francisco, California. Although I knew that the work I was presenting was the result of a profound shift in my beliefs and attitudes as a clinical social worker, it was not clear to me, at that time, what I was recovering from. From my ensuing experiences with mental health service users as employees, colleagues, advocates, employers, friends and family members, I now understand that my recovery is from my own professional stigma about people with mental illnesses. This is a tale about how people with mental illnesses have been, and continue to be, instrumental in my journey of recovery from my stigmatic responses towards them. In telling this story, I will also describe what I consider to be 'best practices' for employing mental health service users within treatment systems, as this is a necessary strategy for addressing professional stigma in the mental health professions.

This story begins in the early 1980s at a forum sponsored by the Community Advisory Board of the Department of Psychiatry at San Francisco General Hospital. The Department had recently become an affiliate of the Department of Psychiatry, University of California, San Francisco, with a mandate to develop programmes, train clinicians and implement research in state-of-the-art practices in community psychiatry. At this time, I was the Chief Psychiatric Social Worker with oversight responsibility for the social work staff of the acute hospital services. I had been appointed as an Assistant Clinical Professor with

59

the university and had a role in teaching the psychiatric residents and students of other mental health disciplines. As an Associate Chief of the Department, I had been involved in developing one of the first clinical case management teams in California. At that time, this was a revolutionary approach for providing comprehensive outpatient treatment to mental health users who experienced multiple hospitalisations.

As a result of its public funding, the department was required to have a Community Advisory Board, made up of volunteers who represented public interests and gave advice to the departmental management. The members of the board were generally enthusiastic about the services and training programmes that the department had been describing to them. However, they also wanted to know what the users of these programmes thought of them. Therefore, a forum was developed at which the mental health services users who had been admitted to the Psychiatric Inpatient Services could share their views of this experience. The large majority of those who spoke had been admitted to an inpatient unit on hold for involuntary treatment.

With courage, clarity and insight, all of the individuals who spoke indicated that they believed that they were poorly treated and received care at a level well below what they would have hoped for. They did not describe physical abuse or maltreatment and, indeed, some indicated that they had been treated with kindness and good intentions. Nevertheless, they indicated that they were not listened to, were not included in decisions about their care and did not feel respected by staff for who they were as people, or what they wanted in their treatment. They also described unnecessary restrictions that abrogated both their rights and their dignity. This was unquestionably the most painful day of my professional career.

My initial response, supported by my professional colleagues, was to explain away this testimony, as being from people who did not represent the general patient population, or with the belief that, as they were being treated involuntarily, they were not able to know what was best for them at the time of their hospitalisation. Even so, as a health professional, I could not be satisfied with my responsibility for delivering services to people who had clearly told me that they found them to be unsatisfactory.

As a result, I began having informal conversations with mental health service users outside of my role as a professional. The more I heard, the more they made sense about what was wrong, not only with hospital care, but with mental health services overall. As important, they had cogent ideas about how to improve mental health services that both made sense, and were more consistent with my professional values than what was often the practice at that time. The response from my professional colleagues, about these conversations, was that I was talking to disgruntled anti-psychiatry advocates who do not understand the purpose or value of the best available treatments. Furthermore, those who had previously been hospitalised, and are now highly functioning and expressing dissatisfaction with the system of care, were probably misdiagnosed initially and are significantly different from the population of people with serious mental illnesses that the hospital served.

Further discussions with these service users, however, indicated that they had experienced significant struggles as a result of serious mental illnesses. These involved multiple hospitalisations including long-term involuntary admissions to the State hospital or locked psychiatric nursing facilities, abuse of drugs and/or alcohol, homelessness, arrests and incarceration, as well as other significant problems resulting from their mental illnesses. In summary, they had once had the exact same characteristics and problems as the highest users of acute inpatient services (Surber et al. 1987). But now they were functioning in community life. Some held jobs and others managed a full, if impoverished, life on entitlements; while all were articulate, outspoken and involved advocates for improved treatment.

This forever changed my understanding about what is possible for people who struggle with serious mental illnesses, even those who experience repeated hospitalisations and multiple problems. Rather than believing the prevailing wisdom of the time that a diagnosis of a serious mental illness required that individuals limit their life expectations, it is quite possible for people with the most serious conditions to live full lives as contributing community members. Furthermore, they have something to teach us about how best to serve them. To me it also meant that actualising this possibility requires professionals to also believe it. Without this belief our subtle and not-so-subtle messages about disabilities and limited functioning will serve to undermine the service users' belief in themselves and risk becoming self-fulfilling prophecies.

It is necessary to note that the term 'recovery' was not used for mental health service users at that time. Having this concept today helps clarify for professionals what it is both necessary and possible to believe in regards to the outcomes for the people we serve.

My questions to service users then became: what helped in changing their lives? How did they get from a life of problems and dysfunction to one of successful community living? Some of those I spoke to said that it was because of their family. Regardless of the troubles that their illnesses and behaviours put on their families, there was someone who loved and never gave up on them. Through this support and belief in them, they were eventually able to accept treatment and begin their recovery. Others said something similar about a mental health professional who maintained a relationship with them, or remained available no matter how much they resisted the help that was offered. Again, this belief that their life could improve resulted in incrementally accepting the support they needed to recover. However, *all* of them said it was their peers that were most helpful. These were people who, like themselves, had struggled with mental illnesses and were recovering from them. These peers provided practical information about how to not only survive, but to thrive with a mental illness. This included practical information about how to obtain community resources and manage the problems they faced in obtaining and using the available treatment and service system. Most importantly, these peers demonstrated that recovery from mental illness is possible and that they too could realise their hopes and dreams.

Through these conversations, I had the opportunity to meet mental health service users who had established peer organisations that were working to improve the lives of people with mental illnesses by developing peer-operated alternative programmes, as an adjunct to the formal treatment system, and by training service users to provide counselling and other services in both peer and professionally managed services. I was so impressed with these efforts that I asked how I could get involved with these peer organisations. I was thanked for my interest and kindly told that if, as a professional, I became an active participant in peer organisations, I would probably take over and they would no longer be what they were intended to be – that is, an organisation of and for mental health service users.

Despite learning so much from mental health services users, I was also becoming increasingly aware of a level of discomfort when talking to them. I felt that I needed to be careful in what I said by not questioning their beliefs or ideas that were different than mine or the prevailing professional wisdom. I was also uncomfortable expressing my own views that I thought might offend them or otherwise interfere with maintaining a 'positive' relationship. However, it eventually occurred to me that I felt no discomfort whatsoever in talking with service users when in a professional relationship. In my role as a clinician, supervisor or programme manager, I could relate with service users with confidence and comfort.

So what was the difference? It was quite simply that I did not know how to relate to people with mental illnesses as equals. This was because, at some level, I experienced them as basically different from me and did not have a way of comfortably relating to them without a professional role. I came to realise that this was a result of my own stigma towards them. How could this be? I saw myself as one whose career was about advocating for people with mental illnesses and building a better service system. I spoke out against stigma, and worked to educate the public about people with mental illnesses and the need for acceptance and tolerance in our communities. But there it was: I was opposed to stigma about those with mental illnesses, and, at the same, perpetuated it through my own beliefs and behaviors.

As a result, I began to see that professional stigma is a reality that undermines the effectiveness of mental health treatment services. It is different than the stigma of the general public that is based on limited understanding of mental illnesses and, often, fear that is based on myths and misperceptions of the people who experience mental illness. Even so, most members of the public are aware of their beliefs and opinions about mentally ill people. Professional stigma is more insidious because it is not recognised. By not acknowledging how experiences, beliefs, and professional dogma undermine the ability to experience service users as equals, mental health providers limit their ability to engage service users in the partnerships necessary to promote recovery.

I now believe that – like recovery from a mental illness – recovery from professional stigma for mental health professionals is an ongoing journey. Resolving it is similar to addressing other prejudices that everyone experiences concerning human differences including race, religion, gender and myriad others. The first step is to acknowledge it. By accepting that we do have stigmatic responses to difference, we can then examine them, be aware when they occur and continuously address them. This is an ongoing process of professional growth. Fortunately for mental health professionals, it is an expectation from our clinical training that we regularly examine responses and reactions in our work in order to continuously improve our ability to establish and maintain effective relationships.

Through my involvement with service users, I have had an increasing appreciation for their value as colleagues within mental health services and the system of care. I also realised that while I might not be able to promote their work in peer-based organisations, I did employ staff in professionally operated organisations, and could develop roles for service users within them. My initial effort was to employ peer counsellors with the Citywide Case Management team for which I had administrative responsibility. From my earlier conversations, I realised that this programme was, at least partly, on the right track. It was a tenet of the programme to never give up on service users who were eligible for this team and to continue to be available to work with them indefinitely; no matter how often they gave up on us (Surber 1994). A theme of the programme was to identify, engage, educate and support family members so that they could better support their family members with a mental illness (Scheidt 1994). However, based on what service users said had helped most, this programme was missing the most important element for promoting recovery: peer support. This led to the employment of peer counselors who worked with case managers to implement the service plans for a high need population with serious mental illnesses.

I now believe that mental health service users are necessary partners with professionals in implementing effective recovery-focused care. This includes service users in roles as direct service providers including as fellow professionals, supervisors, programme managers, leaders, board members and employers of professionals in peer-operated organisations. In addition to being role models for recovery for people in mental health treatment, service users develop peer lead programme models and service strategies in formal treatment programmes based on their experience of what is needed and what is effective for promoting recovery. As important, I believe that the opportunity for professionals to relate to service users as colleagues, outside of their provider role, is necessary for helping professionals, who are not in recovery themselves, to acknowledge and overcome their professional stigma.

There is a growing effort to employ mental health service users in many roles in mental health treatment systems including as direct service providers, support staff, managers and board members. There is also an emerging awareness of the special value of staff who are both clinically trained and have the lived experience of recovery from a mental illness. Nevertheless, many programmes and systems of care struggle to employee service users in meaningful roles in which service-user staff deliver valuable services/supports and are fully accepted by and integrated into the programme. Most clinicians in recovery do not feel comfortable in divulging their diagnosis with a mental illness to either their colleagues or service users, even though this experience can be of value in delivering effective care.

It is my observation that unrecognised professional stigma is often a significant barrier to the successful employment of mental health users and to integrating them, as colleagues, within treatment programmes and systems of care. One issue appears to be that some clinicians do not fully believe in the concept of recovery. Through their training and experience which is often focused on addressing symptoms and disability, many professionals have not had an opportunity to experience service users outside of their professional roles. They are not aware of what is possible when people do recover from mental illnesses.

In addition, some professionals are not aware of the value of peers as colleagues either in terms of how they can be helpful to those treated by the programme or to themselves in learning what they do not know about what can be useful for recovery. As professional stigma is unrecognised, it is expressed through various forms of resistance to employing service users, and to distancing themselves from service user staff after they are hired. It is not uncommon for newly employed service users to feel undermined in their efforts to establish meaningful roles as well as to experience a lack of support, and even hostility, from their professional colleagues. As a result, some programmes that have hired service users are not able to keep these employees for any length of time, and, in others, service users are relegated to meaningless activities. In turn, instead of being an opportunity to overcome professional stigma, the failure to successfully employ peer staff reinforces the professional stigma of clinicians who do not believe in recovery and who do not know the value of service users as colleagues.

The question now becomes: how can professionals make use of the opportunity to address their own stigma through involvement with service-user colleagues, when this stigma undermines their ability to accept and work with service-user providers? Although I am not aware of any methods for directly helping mental health providers in identifying and addressing their professional stigma, I think it can be helpful to learn from what has not worked well to date, and to build upon successful efforts to employ people in recovery.

Determining what does work in employing people in recovery was the focus of a project implemented in Alameda County, California. This informal study interviewed service-user providers, supervisors and managers in both mental health and substance abuse treatment programmes that served people with dual disorders (with a co-occurring substance abuse and mental health diagnosis). As substance abuse services have long employed people in recovery (and not infrequently in dual recovery) to deliver treatment services, this provided an opportunity to learn what is successful in employing people in recovery in programmes that have a history of doing so, as well as in services for which this was a relatively new idea. The report from this project describes several 'best practices' for successfully integrating service users as peer providers in behavioral health programs (PEERS 2004). These strategies are described as follows:

- User Training (and Certification) – The lived experience of recovery is not sufficient to succeed as a treatment provider and some training is necessary to prepare people for the roles they will be fulfilling. There are now peer provider training programmes in many communities (often designed and delivered by peer organisations), and some jurisdictions provide a certification as peer specialist.
- Prepare Professionals and Other Staff – Professionals must be involved in the decision and process for bringing in colleagues that will affect their work. They do have legitimate questions and concerns that need to be addressed. Working through these issues prior to employing peers can help with successful integration of new roles.
- Clear Job Descriptions – Providing a clear understanding of the role to be implemented along with measures of success and lines of accountability helps both the peer and professional staff know what is expected of each other and defines expectations for collaboration.
- Employ People with Ability to do the Job – As with any position, it is necessary hire a person who is capable of and interested in doing the job at hand. Being in recovery and being certified as a peer specialist are no more sufficient for successful employment than is holding a degree or professional licensure.
- Same Rights and Responsibilities for all Staff – Peer and professional staff enjoy all of the same rights and are held accountable for the same responsibilities. This includes meeting responsibilities for confidentiality, punctuality and for legal and regulatory requirements. It also means access to records as necessary, participation in staff meetings and other organisational events, including celebrations.
- Separate Employee and Service-User Roles – When employed, service users are at the organisation to do a job. They are to be treated the same as any other staff with regards to any health problem or disability they may experience. Maintaining the separation of user and employee roles can be challenging for both service user and professional staff who are used to relating within a treatment relationship and not as colleagues. This is particularly important when service users are employed within an organisation from which they receive treatment.
- Ongoing Opportunities to Share Expertise – Professional and peer providers have experiences and expertise that, when shared, can improve the ability of all staff to deliver more effective care. It is helpful to

create forums, such as staff meetings, case conferences, in-service training and group supervision in which the experiences and expertise of everyone is offered, acknowledged and accepted as an opportunity to learn.

- Offer Reasonable Accommodation – In employing any person with a self-disclosed disability, it is necessary to provide reasonable accommodations that allow for successful completion of the work. For mental health service users, some accommodations have included part-time employment and flexible work hours to meet individual needs.
- User Staff Support Groups – Service-user employees can feel isolated in a programme in which most staff are professionals and other non-service-user employees. Support groups for service-user employees within a programme or agency or between organisations can offer support and the sharing of solutions to problems that arise in their roles.
- Provide Adequate Supervision – No amount of training can prepare service users for the issues they will face in working as providers. In addition, unlike professionals, they have not experienced coursework and internships that provide acculturation to these work settings. This speaks to the need for additional supervision time for service-user staff. This can be experienced as a burden by supervisory staff, but could be considered to be a reasonable accommodation that is necessary for successful employment of a population experiencing a mental health disability.
- Encourage Employment of Professionals in Recovery – In some treatment settings, professionals who acknowledge that they are in recovery are considered to be very valuable employees. In addition to their clinical training and experiences with a mental illness, which can be of help with the people they treat, this background can also be of support in bridging the differences between professional and peer staff within the programme. To encourage professionals to be more open about their treatment histories, it can be helpful to include as a desired qualification for all positions, experience with recovery from a mental illness.

Overall, the 'best practices' for employing service users in mental health agencies are similar to good personnel practices for everyone.

There is currently a worldwide effort to transform mental health treatment through the establishment of recovery-focused systems of care. It has been suggested that, to be successful, this requires transforming the staff who provide these services. In recovery-focused services, providers must be able to partner with those they serve, and work to support them in identifying and implementing their individual journey of recovery. This will not be effective with professionals who do not believe in recovery or who are not aware of their own stigmatic responses and how they can interfere with building these necessary partnerships.

My own recovery from professional stigma is an ongoing process that has been inspired, supported, cajoled and/or pounded into me by many people in recovery from mental illnesses in numerous roles. Over these years, service users have become my best teachers. But first I had to identify and begin to address my stigma, so that I was able to hear them.

References

PEERS (2004) *What Works?: Employment of People in Recovery in Alameda County Behavioral Health Care Services* (unpublished report by Peers Envisioning and Engaging in Recovery, commissioned by The Alameda County Behavioral Health Care Services Consumer Employment Opportunities Committee and prepared with Robert W. Surber, Consultation in Behavioral Health, San Francisco, CA).

Scheidt, S. (1994). 'Engaging Families and Natural Support Systems', in R. W. Surber (ed.). *Clinical Case Management: A Guide to Comprehensive Treatment of Serious Mental Illness* (Sage: Thousand Oaks, CA).

Surber, R., Winkler, E., Monteleone, M., Havassy, B., Goldfinger, S. and Hopkin, J. (1987). 'Characteristics of High Users of Acute Psychiatric In-patient Services', *Hospital and Community Psychiatry*, XXXVIII, 10.

Surber, R. W. (1994). 'An Approach to Care', in R. W. Surber (ed.). *Clinical Case Management: A Guide to Comprehensive Treatment of Serious Mental Illness* (Sage: Thousand Oaks, CA).

5

Developing Successful Recovery-Oriented Mental Health Services

Jed Boardman and Geoff Shepherd

Introduction: a rationale for recovery-oriented services

In this chapter, we describe a project which has examined the principles and concepts of recovery, and looked at ways in which mental health practices and services could be orientated to facilitate recovery in people who use these services. There has been a developing body of literature on the research evidence for the value of recovery principles. Many such sources (Warner 2009, 2010) have given a particular emphasis to the value and importance of optimism about outcome in psychosis, and the value of empowerment and of productive social roles such as employment. There is also a vast literature on the experience of service users and their own accounts of their recovery journeys, their experiences of mental health services and what they require from these services (Repper and Perkins 2003, Slade 2009).

The opportunity afforded to such developments by current mental health policy in certain countries is considerable, not only in the United Kingdom (UK), but also in other countries such as Australia (Australian Government 2005), the USA (Department of Health and Human Services 2003), New Zealand (Mental Health Commission 1998) and Ireland (Mental Health Commission, 2005). In the UK, there has been support from major mental health professional organisations (Royal College of Psychiatrists 2007 and 2009, College of Occupational Therapists 2006, British Psychological Society 2000, Royal College of Nursing 2009, South London and Maudsley NHS Foundation Trust and South West London and St George's Mental Health NHS Trust 2010).

In the UK in the last ten years, Mental Health Policy and General Health Policy have supported the ideas of recovery (Boardman et al. 2010). The last Labour government's mental health strategy, *New Horizons*, placed recovery in a central position in future developments (DOH 2009). With the advent of a new government, the 2009 policy document has now been replaced by a new policy paper *No Health without Mental Health: A Cross-Government Mental Health Outcomes Strategy for People of All Ages* (DOH 2011), which now forms the cornerstone of mental health policy for the new Conservative-Liberal coalition. This document retains recovery as a core element of its overall strategy. The second of its six objectives is 'More people with mental health problems will recover' which states,

> *More people who develop mental health problems will have a good quality of life – greater ability to manage their own lives, stronger social relationships, a greater sense of purpose, the skills they need for living and working, improved chances in education, better employment rates and a suitable and stable place to live.*

(DOH 2011)

What has not yet happened in any systematic way is the translation of the ideas and principles of recovery into practice and the delivery of mental health services. This translation of principles into practice has been a central concern of our work. Although we have come across many examples of good practice in the area of recovery, many mental health service providers both in the UK and internationally have made little progress and there is no clear guidance, consensus or strategy as to how comprehensive services which are based on recovery principles might best be developed. One aim of our project was to develop ways in which these omissions could be rectified.

Recovery – a definition

Anthony has given one of the most commonly accepted definitions of recovery, which may be paraphrased as 'living a life beyond illness':

> *a deeply personal, unique process of changing ones attitudes, values, feelings goals, skills, and/or roles. It is a way of living a satisfying, hopeful and contributing life even with the limitations caused by illness. Recovery involves the development of new meaning and purpose in one's life as one grows beyond the catastrophic effects of mental illness.*

(Anthony, 1993)

Analysis of service-user accounts of their recovery journeys suggests that three concepts make up the central aspects of recovery

(Repper and Perkins 2003): *hope* (sustaining motivation and supporting expectations of an individually fulfilled life), *agency* (recovering a sense of personal control) and *opportunity* (using circumstances to gain favourable ends).

Hope is a central aspect of recovery and some would say that recovery is impossible without hope. Essentially this means that if an individual cannot see the possibility of a decent future for themselves, then it is difficult if not impossible to motivate themselves towards the future.

Agency, in the sense used here, is concerned with who is in control and refers to service users taking control over their own problems, their life and their future. This implies taking control over such matters as the way they understand what has happened to them, their problems and the help they receive, what they do in their lives, their dreams and their ambitions. This also involves self-management and self-determination, choice and responsibility.

The third concept, *opportunity*, links to the concept of social inclusion or participation in a wider society. Social inclusion is important for recovery as people with mental health problems and disabilities in general wish to be part of our communities, to be valued members of those communities, to have access to the opportunities that exist in those communities, and to have the opportunity to contribute to those communities (Boardman et al. 2010).

The problems of implementation

A key concern of many attempting to implement recovery is the often-heard statement from workers in mental health services that they are now 'doing recovery'. It is clear that professionals do not 'do recovery' and recovery cannot be implemented by services. We know that recovery has been formulated by and for service users, to describe their own experiences: it is service users who 'do recovery', not professionals.

Nevertheless, professionals (and mental health services) can influence recovery and recovery journeys: they can impede them (as has often been the case) but they can also facilitate them. It is this idea of facilitating recovery that has become a central focus of the Recovery Project (supported in the Centre for Mental Health, London) described in this chapter. If recovery is to have an impact, then professionals and others working in mental health services need to understand what recovery means and, in partnership with service users and others, actively support processes supportive to recovery across services. This requires giving attention to changing the way services operate, changing the structure and the culture of service organisations, in order for them to become 'recovery-orientated'. This project examined what services need to do to achieve this. It focused on two main questions: how can we put the ideas of recovery into practice and what are the challenges to this?

The centre for mental health project: 'supporting recovery'

To support the project, we assembled a Steering Group representing five National Health Service (NHS) provider organisations (called Health Trusts in England) and their local partners who had already made significant progress towards implementing more recovery-oriented practices. The group consisted of clinical experts in this field, service users and people from the major mental health charities.

We produced an initial Briefing Paper '*Making Recovery a Reality*' (Shepherd, Boardman and Slade 2008), which summarised the key principles of recovery and how these link to practices and services, the common objections to recovery and some of the possible problems of implementation.

We then ran a series of local workshops in the five NHS Trusts during 2008 and 2009, each examining a different area of organisational change that we thought necessary to address in order to move towards more recovery-oriented services. The workshops were attended by more than 300 people including a range of health and social care professionals, managers and representatives from local independent organizations, with extensive input from service users and carers (Chandler 2010).

The output of these workshops was published as a short document – 'Implementing Recovery. A New Framework for Organisational Change' (Sainsbury Centre for Mental Health 2009) which set out ten key challenges for organisational change (see Box 5.2 below).

What are the implication for mental health services?

What are the implications of the ideas and principles of recovery described above for mental health services? We already know that we can be more optimistic about the outcomes of psychoses, that empowerment of people with mental health problems improves outcomes and that there are well-tested ways to get people with severe mental illness into work (Warner 2009 and 2010). But we need to go further than this. There needs to be a focus on services in which decisions are taken collaboratively with service users, and services which aim to assist people with mental health problems into productive roles. There also needs to be

- Increased awareness of the impact of practices and procedures on people's sense of control
- Greater emphasis placed on encouraging people to find their own *meaning* in events (not simple 'psycho-education')
- Explicit attempts to reduce the traditional power differences between those using the service and those providing it
- Recognition of the value of 'experts-by-experience'
- Greater emphasis on *social goals*, rather than only *clinical outcomes*
- Redefinition of professional roles
- Recognition that professionals can act as 'carriers of hope'.

Practise, services and culture

From the workshops, needs for change were identified in the following areas:

- *practice* (staff and professional training),
- *service organisation and delivery*,
- *culture of services*.

These areas of change are not independent of each other: the three areas should be addressed in parallel. Practices and services and what they deliver should be based on the best available evidence.

Practice – role of professionals

This has been covered in more detail elsewhere (Shepherd, Boardman, and Slade 2008, Boardman et al. 2010), but the basic changes need to be

- A shift in the relationship to one emphasising partnership, along the lines of that between a *coach* and an *expert by experience*
- A shift away from 'doing to' to providing resources to facilitate self-management, with professionals being seen as *on tap, not on top*
- The provision of hope in a realistic and pragmatic way
- A shift in the central objectives to social outcomes, including housing, employment, education, participation in mainstream community and leisure activities.

Box 5.1 Ten Top Tips for recovery-oriented practice (Shepherd, Boardman, and Slade 2008)

After each interaction, ask yourself 'did I ...'

1. actively listen to help the person make sense of their mental health problems?
2. help the person identify and prioritise their personal goals for recovery – not my professional goals?
3. demonstrate a belief in the person's existing strengths and resources in relation to the pursuit of these goals?
4. identify examples from my own 'lived experience', or that of other service users, which inspire and validate their hopes?
5. pay particular attention to the importance of goals which take the person out of the 'sick role' and enable them actively to contribute to the lives of others?
6. identify non-mental health resources – friends, contacts, organisations – relevant to the achievement of their goals?
7. encourage self-management of mental health problems (by providing information, reinforcing existing coping strategies and other strategies)?
8. discuss what the person wants in terms of therapeutic interventions, for example psychological treatments, alternative therapies, joint crisis planning, respecting their wishes wherever possible?
9. behave at all times so as to convey an attitude of respect for the person and a desire for an equal partnership in working together, indicating a willingness to 'go the extra mile'?
10. while accepting that the future is uncertain and setbacks will happen, continue to express support for the possibility of achieving these self-defined goals – maintaining hope and positive expectations?

For professionals, we devised a list of Ten Top Tips for recovery-oriented practice (see Box 5.1) which have proved useful in getting the practice changes over to professionals. They have been readily taken up by colleagues and can be used for training.

Services and culture – changing experience, changing values

Not only changes to clinical practice, but organisational changes are necessary to move services to become more recovery-orientated. The ideas of recovery must go right through the organisation, influencing it at every level. First and foremost, there needs to be a fundamental *change in the quality of day-to-day interactions*. Every interaction, by every member of staff, should confirm recovery principles and promote recovery values. This means introducing comprehensive, *user-led education and training programmes* for all staff, across all professions and at all levels. This requires a supply of *trained and supported service users* to act as the 'champions of change'. To provide this, we suggest the creation of a *Recovery Education Unit* in each Trust, run by user-educators, linked to the Trust's development strategy and to local education providers, in order to ensure standards.

However, training alone will not be enough. Recovery values need to become *embedded into every management process*, including recruitment, supervision, management and appraisal, and operational policies. It must be embedded in the language of the organisation such as in its mission statements, straplines, policies and other official documents. This means *leadership* from senior levels, combined with the effective use of information.

Within the organisation, a greater emphasis on recovery should lead to increased individualisation of care, with, among others, more shared decision-making (for example, regarding treatments) and use of individual budgets. There also needs to be a revision of the guidelines and procedures for *risk assessment and management*, which should be more open, transparent and increasingly involve the service user in a partnership approach.

Making these changes will inevitably lead to a fundamental *review of skill-mix and professional/user balance* within the workforce. We should consider a radical transformation, aiming for perhaps half of care delivery by appropriately trained and supported 'peer specialists' (Ashcraft and Anthony 2005, Chinman et al. 2008, Repper and Carter 2010). These developments have implications for recruitment processes and for the running of Human Resource and Occupational Health Departments. In addition, we will also need to *support staff (and carers) in their recovery journeys*; valuing their 'lived experience' and the contribution that this can make to their professional roles.

Finally, the changes that are needed will mean *opening up the organisation*, turning it around to be outward, instead of inward-facing and developing partnerships with non-mental health agencies, particularly in housing and employment, so that these become the central focus, not secondary additions. Supporting people using the service to build a life *'beyond illness'* means achieving not just integration in the community, but inclusion within it.

All these points are summarised in Box 5.2 as the Ten key challenges for organisational change.

Box 5.2 Ten key challenges for organisational change (Sainsbury Centre for Mental Health, 2009)

1. Changing the nature of day-to-day interactions and the quality of experience
2. Delivering comprehensive, user-led education and training programmes
3. Establishing a 'Recovery Education Unit' to drive the programmes forward
4. Ensuring organisational commitment, creating the 'culture'
5. Increasing 'personalisation' and choice
6. Transforming the workforce
7. Changing the way we approach risk assessment and management
8. Redefining user involvement
9. Supporting staff in their recovery journey
10. Increasing opportunities for building a life 'beyond illness'.

Developing the approach – organisational change

The key challenges shown in Box 5.2 can provide a starting point for organisational development, as they summarise the main headings for a ten-point plan to develop a recovery-orientated organisation. However, this needs to be tested out; so, in 2010, we began a new implementation project in 29 NHS Mental Health provider organisations: the *Im*plementing *R*ecovery *O*rganisational *C*hange (ImROC) Project. We have produced a methodology to support this (Shepherd, Boardman and Burns 2010) which is designed to assist organisational change and the commissioning of services, and to improve process and outcomes.

The methodology incorporates a simple two-phase process:

Phase 1 – Developing the 'vision' and benchmarking

In the first part of the process, the stakeholders try to get to grips with the complexities of the new ideas and assess the stage of progression of the main, local NHS provider on each of the ten key organisational challenges using a simple, three-stage classification:

Engagement – The organisation is clearly engaged in its intent to deliver recovery-oriented services. Plans have been made but with little progress as yet.

Development – Action is being taken with some evidence of significant developments in practice, policy and culture. Good progress is being made in delivering recovery-oriented services in some areas, but this is not consistent throughout the organisation.

Transformation – The vision for achieving significant change has been fully realised. The necessary policy processes and practice to deliver a recovery-orientated service is embedded at every level of the organisation. There are processes in place to achieve continuous improvements based on learning from ongoing review.

This assessment provides a summary of the current situation and could be used for benchmarking purposes, although the primary purpose of this part of the process is to develop an understanding of the concepts and their implications for organisational change. This part of the method therefore comprises discussions at a local level to understand the current situation and the status of the provider with regard to each of the organisational challenges. Providers and other local stakeholders are asked to draw on their different perspectives to come to a shared consensus.

Phase 2 – Developing the strategy, monitoring and review

After completing this general assessment, the provider and others then move to the second part of the process. In this, the main NHS provider, commissioners and other stakeholders jointly agree on the priorities for organisational change. They need to prioritise action in a small number of areas and agree on some *SMART* (Specific, Measurable, Agreed-upon, Realistic, Time-based) goals to define the targets and monitor outcomes. Actions to achieve these goals can then be implemented, their progress monitored and evaluated, the goals reset and then further monitored in an iterative process. This 'Plan-Do-Study-Act' cycle is recommended as the most effective process for producing sustained organisational change (Iles and Sutherland 2001).

Each of the ten key organisational challenges presents a potentially substantial agenda for organisational change, and together they open up opportunities to transform services in ways that are much more consistent with the priorities of service users and their families. However, it is unlikely (and unrealistic) that all the ten challenges can be addressed immediately; the organisation change strategy will need to be implemented over a number of years. The priorities for organisational change jointly agreed at any one time should be limited to a realistic number, possibly no more than five at one time. Clearly all local services are different and all will start from a different point in their development of these innovatory services.

Once there is agreement about the service level goals to be achieved and a clear description of the actions, timescales and responsibilities for achieving them, progress can be tracked. To assist with setting and monitoring specific targets, we have developed a series of examples of service-level indicators and potential data sources for each of the organisational challenges (Shepherd, Boardman and Burns 2010). Such examples are intended to be illustrative, rather than prescriptive, and alternative indicators may be substituted, or added if they reflect better the chosen targets. Providers, service users and commissioners should determine locally which indicators they are going to use and how ambitious the targets will be. This gives them maximum flexibility, within a clear and comprehensive framework.

The methodology described here involves a constructive process of 'co-production' between local providers and commissioners, in partnership with service users and carers, which aims to transform services through the development of the jointly agreed key areas of recovery-oriented practice. A key element driving this transformation will be the joint work of local systems, setting priorities, agreeing on goals and contracts and then moving the process forward.

Importantly, there is a need to avoid being too rigid and formulaic as this runs the risk of locking local providers and commissioners into a rigid view of how these essentially innovative developments should proceed. We believe that our approach offers a flexible means of delivering organisational change towards more recovery-orientated services. The experience gained from working with the organisations involved in the ImROC project will provide further evidence as to how services can best be encouraged to make genuine, evidence-based progress towards delivering authentic recovery-orientated services.

The *Im*plementing *R*ecovery *O*rganisational *C*hange (ImROC) Project

This project is aimed at assisting English NHS mental health services, together with their local independent sector partners and user and carer groups, to develop recovery-orientated services. The project is funded by the Department of Health and is being delivered by a partnership between the Mental Health Network of the NHS Confederation and the Centre for Mental Health. In addition to the two chapter authors, the project team also consists of Rachel Perkins and Julie Repper. We are also supported by a group of service-user trainers. We are using the methodology described above.

More than 30 provider organisations (mostly NHS Mental Health Trusts) in England applied to be a part of the programme and 29 are now taking part. The 29 provider organisations were grouped into three categories, according to their progress with regard to the ten key challenges for organisational change and their corresponding need for support.

Demonstration sites (n=6). These were judged to have already made significant or outstanding progress regarding the 'ten key challenges' and successfully embedding recovery principles into the organisation. They will receive up to ten days' expert consultancy on topics of their choice.

Pilot sites (n=6). These had made some progress in addressing the key challenges and 'embedding' the principles, but less than the Demonstration sites. They showed good, local partnership working and were keen to develop their services. They will receive 25 days' consultancy with support from expert peer trainers to develop local, user-led training initiatives. While some direct training will be undertaken, the emphasis will be on building local capacity.

Network sites (n=17). These were not as advanced as either the Demonstration or the Pilot sites in terms of progress against the key challenges and/or organisational 'embedding'.

All 29 sites will have the opportunity to send 6–8 people to local 'Learning Sets', consisting of six one-day workshops conducted over two years. These will be mixed groups, consisting of Demonstration, Pilot and Network sites and will provide the opportunity to share ideas and experiences and to gain support from others who are working on similar issues.

The work with the sites began in 2011 and preliminary discussions have revealed a number of common themes that the Mental Health Trusts have been working on, which include

- Support for development of local user/staff learning about recovery, with local users and staff working together with 'peer experts'
- Active consideration of plans to establish 'Recovery Colleges'
- The need for work to inform senior managers (usually at the Board level) and key clinical leaders, including psychiatrists, psychologists and professional leads.
- The need to review key policies and procedures such as care planning documentation and risk assessment and management
- Developing training for peer specialists
- Working with carers.

Conclusions

Recovery is probably the most important current new direction for mental health services. It represents the convergence of a number of ideas (empowerment, self-management, disability rights, social inclusion and rehabilitation) under a single heading that offers a new direction for mental health services. The ideas of recovery, developed from the accounts of service users' own experience, have influenced thinking in mental health services across the world and have been supported at national policy level in several countries. They can form the guiding principles for our future mental health services, offer a means to transform the way we organise mental health services and to improve the quality of local services in order to support service users to lead meaningful and productive lives. The key challenges identified in the current project form a basis to begin working in partnership with service users and with carers to change the practice, delivery and culture of mental health services. By doing so, we can begin to address the limitations and barriers for people with mental health problems to live in hope, exercise greater choice and control and to have access to a greater range of opportunities to live a life that they value and choose.

References

Ashcraft, L. and Anthony, W. A. (2005). 'A Story of Transformation: An Agency Fully Embraces Recovery', *Behavioural Healthcare Tomorrow*, XIV, 12–22.

Australian Government (2003). *Australian Health Ministers National Mental Health Plan 2003–2008* (Australian Government: Canberra).

Boardman, J., Currie, A., Killaspy, H. and Mezey, G. (2010). *Social Inclusion and Mental Health* (London: RCPsych Publications).

British Psychological Society Division of Clinical Psychology (2000). *Recent Advances in Understanding Mental Illness and Psychotic Experiences* (British Psychological Society: Leicester).

Chandler, R. (2010). *Making Recovery a Reality: A Lived Experience Perspective of the Sainsbury Centre for Mental Health Workshops* (London: Sainsbury Centre for Mental Health).

Chinman, M., Lucksted, A., Gresen, R., Davis, M., Losonczy, M., Sussner, B. and Martone, L. (2008). 'Early Experiences of Employing Consumer-Providers in the VA', *Psychiatric Services*, LIX, 1315–21.

College of Occupational Therapists (2006). *Recovering Ordinary Lives: The Strategy for Occupational Therapy in Mental Health Services 2007–2017* (College of Occupational Therapists: London).

Department of Health (DOH) (2011). *No Health without Mental Health. A Cross-Government Mental Health Outcomes Strategy for People of All Ages*, Mental Health Division (Department of Health: London).

Department of Health (DOH) (2009). *New Horizons: A Shared Vision for Mental Health* (Mental Health Division, London).

Department of Health and Human Services (2003). *Achieving the Promise: Transforming Mental Health Care in America. President's New Freedom Commission on Mental Health*, pub. no. SMA–03–3832 (Rockville, Maryland, US).

Iles, V. and Sutherland, K. (2001). 'Organisational Change – A Review for Health Care Managers, Professionals and Researchers' (National Co-ordinating Centre for NHS Service Delivery and Organisation (NCCSDO), London School of Hygiene and Tropical Medicine).

Mental Health Commission (1998). *Blueprint for Mental Health Services in New Zealand* (Mental Health Commission: Wellington NZ).

Mental Health Commission (2005). *A Vision for a Recovery Model in Irish Mental Health Services* (Mental Health Commission: Dublin).

Repper, J. and Carter, T. (2010). *Using Personal Experience to Support Others with Similar Difficulties. A Review of the Literature on Peer Support in Mental Health Services* (London: Together).

Repper, J. and Perkins, R. (2003). *Social Inclusion and Recovery* (London: Balliere Tindall).

Royal College of Nursing (2009). *Socially Inclusive Practice for Nurses* (London: Royal College of Nursing).

Royal College of Psychiatrists (2009). *Mental Health and Social Inclusion. Making Psychiatry and Mental Health Services Fit for the 21st Century* (London: Royal College of Psychiatrists).

Royal College of Psychiatrists/Social Care Institute for Excellence/Care Services Improvement Partnership (2007). *A Common Purpose: Recovery in Future Mental Health Services* (Social Care Institute for Excellence: London), http://www.scie.org.uk/publications/positionpapers/pp08.pdf, date accessed 14 June 2011.

Sainsbury Centre for Mental Health (2009). 'Implementing Recovery – A New Framework for Organisational Change', position paper (London: Sainsbury Centre for Mental Health).

Shepherd, G., Boardman, J. and Slade, M. (2008). *Making Recovery a Reality* (London: Sainsbury Centre for Mental Health).

Shepherd, G., Boardman, J. and Burns, M. (2010). *Implementing Recovery. A Methodology for Organisational Change* (London: Sainsbury Centre for Mental Health).

Slade, M. (2009). *Personal Recovery and Mental Illness: A Guide for Mental Health Professional* (Cambridge: Cambridge University Press).

South London and Maudsley NHS Foundation Trust and South West London and St George's Mental Health NHS Trust (2010). 'Recovery is for All. Hope, Agency and Opportunity in Psychiatry'. A Position Statement by Consultant Psychiatrists (London: SLAM/SWLSTG).

Warner, R. (2009). 'Recovery from Schizophrenia and the Recovery Model', *Current Opinion in Psychiatry*, XXII, 374–80.

Warner, R. (2010). 'Does the Scientific Evidence Support the Recovery Model', *The Psychiatrist*, XXXIV, 3–5.

Part II

Social Inclusion and Employment

6
Designing Policies to Foster the Community Inclusion of People in Recovery

Larry Davidson, Elizabeth Flanagan and Thomas Styron

For the purposes of this chapter, we would like to begin by drawing an important distinction between community *integration* and community *inclusion*, explaining why we have chosen the latter for the task at hand. Community integration is the notion that has been used more often in the history of community mental health, and its use reflects the limited success of that movement. Briefly stated, community integration refers to the process of assisting a person to become re-engaged in community life, and the reciprocal process of assisting a community to accept and welcome back persons who have been extruded from community life, *once the person's condition has been resolved*. In this sense, community integration can refer equally well to offenders returning to the community from prison or immigrants becoming acculturated to the community they have chosen to adopt, and be adopted by. In each of these cases, what marked the person as different and accounted for his or her need *to be* integrated (what caused his or her exclusion or alienation in the first place) is no longer present. In the case of mental illness, this has meant be cured of your illness first, recover from or overcome the symptoms and deficits associated with the illness first, and then we will welcome you back within our community. The problem with applying this model to mental illnesses is that we do not yet have a cure for these conditions.

Community inclusion, on the other hand, comes primarily from the disability community, and assumes that certain conditions will not go away, at least for the foreseeable future, if not for the remainder of the person's life. For such people whose conditions cannot yet be resolved, a community integration paradigm makes little sense, as they do not want to wait – nor should they be made to wait – to recover from or overcome their disability in order to enjoy all of the rights and responsibilities of full community membership. The community inclusion paradigm argues instead that people with long-term disabilities – including people with long-term *psychiatric* disabilities – should be accepted and welcomed by their communities as they are, with whatever conditions they may have, without having to be cured, fixed, or otherwise made to conform to selected societal norms first. The prototype for community inclusion is thus people with a range of physical disabilities for whom accommodations have been successfully developed, such as people who use wheelchairs to compensate for mobility impairments, people who use Braille or service dogs to compensate for visual impairments, and people who use sign language and visual cues (for example, for phones and doorbells) to compensate for auditory impairments. In these cases, the community bears a share of the responsibility for accommodating the person's disability, for making its own changes (for example installing handrails in bathrooms and Braille signs on elevators) in order to facilitate the person's full access to and involvement in community life. It is the person's responsibility to learn, or figure out, how to compensate for the disability and to take advantage of the accommodations provided in order to pursue a full and contributing life.

Since the field of psychiatry has yet to discover or develop a cure for serious mental illness, and since the treatments that currently exist are extremely limited in their effectiveness even in containing the illness, we argue in this chapter that community inclusion represents a more appropriate and promising approach for persons living with serious mental illnesses than the traditional approach of community integration. Consistent with at least some camps within the international Mental Health User/Consumer/Survivor Movement, we argue that the adoption of a disability paradigm opens up new opportunities and creates access to a range of new and more effective supports for people who have yet to recover from the illness. In response to the remaining camps within this Movement who reject a disability paradigm, it is important to add that adoption of a community inclusion paradigm need not consign a person to a life of dependency and disability. It does not indicate or require a giving up of hope or effort towards full recovery. Rather, it is based on research and accumulated clinical experience that suggests that recovery is more likely to be promoted by the person's efforts to reclaim his or her life despite symptoms or impairments, rather than by waiting for the symptoms or impairments to disappear. In other words, a person is more likely to go from learning how to live fully *with* a disability to no longer being disabled at all ('full' recovery) than to go directly from being ill to being well. In terms of (albeit imperfect) medical analogies, serious and prolonged mental illnesses are more like chronic illnesses such as asthma than like acute illnesses such as the flu or an infection.

How, then, to design social policies to foster the community inclusion of persons with serious and prolonged psychiatric disabilities? How to create accommodations, or make what are called 'environmental modifications', to facilitate the inclusion of people who are 'in recovery' with a serious mental illness? We use 'in recovery' in this context to refer to that form of 'recovery' introduced and advocated for by the User/Consumer/Survivor movement, which we distinguish from the traditional medical/psychiatric concept of 'recovering from' the disorder. Being 'in recovery' refers to living a safe, dignified, gratifying, self-determined life in the face of an ongoing mental illness, rather than to no longer experiencing the signs, symptoms, and impairments associated with the disorder. In this way, being in recovery parallels the notion of living with a psychiatric disability, with the added connotation that the person has taken charge of his or her life and is actively pursuing ways of managing and compensating for the disability (rather than living a life of despair or resignation). Readers who are interested in learning more about this distinction between recovering from and being in recovery are referred to a previous publication on this topic (Davidson and Roe 2007).

We suggest that there are at least three different foci for policies to foster community inclusion for people 'in recovery'. The first of these is a focus on the mental health system itself, and on how it can better promote community inclusion through the services and supports it offers. The second focus is on the interface between the mental health system and the broader community, and on innovative strategies the mental health system can adopt to make this interface more porous in both directions. The third and final focus is on the broader community, the locus of the inclusion to be achieved, and on how it can better facilitate and accommodate the involvement of people with psychiatric disabilities. We will take each in turn.

Policies focused on the mental health system

In terms of the mental health system, it is an unfortunate reality that most mental health services currently pose more of an obstacle to community inclusion than facilitate it. This is due to a number of factors, but stems primarily from the history of institutionalisation and its effects, leaving a legacy of prejudice and discrimination against persons with serious mental illnesses that has lingered within community-based service systems. This legacy can be found on three levels within the mental health system: the institutional level, the level of the individual client or service recipient, and the level of individual providers.

By 'institutional level', we refer to the fact that many of the current policies of mental health systems inhibit rather than promote the community inclusion of people in recovery. Some of these may be attributed to the legacy of secrecy and neutrality fostered by the psychodynamic paradigm, which has created rigid and hierarchical boundaries between practitioners and their patients or clients. While intended to protect the person's privacy and allow for projection of the person's internal conflicts onto a practitioner well-prepared and trained to make therapeutic use of these projections, these boundaries have instead created a static, two-class system in which people seeking services are made to feel inferior to their care providers and often end up viewing themselves as having nothing of value to offer in interpersonal relationships – relationships which then come to be characterised as one-directional (Davidson, Stayner and Haglund 1998). Rather than serving as the bridge to mutual relationships in the broader community that the psychotherapeutic relationship was originally intended to be, such asymmetrical relationships serve instead to keep people stuck within the mental health system, convinced that they are not fully people and that they have nothing to offer others as a basis for mutuality. A related, if unintended, result of this attitude is having separate staff and patient/client bathrooms in outpatient settings – reminiscent of the 'White' and 'Coloured' only bathrooms and drinking fountains in the segregated American South prior to the 1960s – reinforcing the message that people with mental illnesses are fundamentally different from (and less than) those without.

Other policies that serve as impediments to inclusion are based on the problematic assumption described above that people need to be cured of, or recovered from, a mental illness prior to resuming other social roles (more valued than that of mental patient) such as student, worker, friend, lover, tenant, neighbour, congregant or voter. Within the service setting, this assumption has led mental health practitioners to view their patients/clients as incompetent to make their own decisions, set their own goals, or pursue their own dreams and aspirations, until and unless they have recovered. One of the several important things missing from such an approach is any recognition that making one's own decisions, setting one's own goals, and pursuing one's own aspirations are all crucial components of the recovery process itself. By disallowing, at worst, or discouraging, at best, the person from making his or her own choices and pursuing his or her own interests, mental health services have unfortunately relegated the person to and kept him or her trapped within a passive, dependant, disabled, and despondent role. If I need to 'get better' before I can reclaim a life in the community, and yet I have to take steps towards reclaiming a life in the community as a core component *of* 'getting better', then I become and remain stuck; a fate we have tragically seen befall generations of individuals with serious mental illnesses.

To reverse these destructive practices, policies focused on promoting community inclusion would therefore begin with examining the status and role of the person in recovery within the mental health system itself. We, within the mental health system, cannot reasonably expect the community to reject stigma and discrimination against people in recovery if we cannot get our own house in order first. Doing so will require opening up opportunities for people with mental illnesses to take on a variety of proactive and constructive roles in reviewing, monitoring, evaluating, governing, improving, staffing, and otherwise giving their input into the mental health system. People in recovery will be invited to participate in, and eventually will comprise the majority of, boards of directors, governing bodies, advisory councils, steering committees, quality improvement teams, and other workgroups focused on designing and improving the functioning of mental health agencies and systems. They will be offered the opportunities and supports to become effective mental health practitioners, evaluators, and researchers as well as advocates, and their contributions will be increasingly valued as services and systems become more responsive as a result.

An excellent example of the kinds of steps involved in increasing the involvement of people in recovery in these and other ways can be found in the substantial amount of user input and participation recently encouraged by the policy unit of the Royal College of Psychiatrists in England (Fitch et al. 2008). Experiences such as these within the mental health system have the added benefit of preparing people in recovery for similar roles in the broader community.

Once established at the organisational level, such a framework of inclusion can then extend to the level of the individual service recipient. Increasing self-determination and self-direction at the level of the individual requires people in recovery to be placed in charge of their own treatment, or recovery, plan. Rather than remaining the passive recipient of the ameliorative efforts of caring others (Davidson 1997) who are limited to adhering (or not) to the prescriptions formulated by experts, people in recovery will need to become active, and leading, participants in formulating their own action plans for their unique recovery journeys (Tondora et al. 2005). Like health care consumers for other conditions, they will need to become educated about their condition and the options of treatments and other interventions available to them, and empowered to make their own decisions about which of these resources will be most useful to them in pursuing their life goals.

Experience suggests that when people in recovery become active in these ways, they become much more likely to identify goals for their recovery plans in the various domains of community life such as housing, jobs, education, and social and recreational activities than when limited to a subordinate role in treatment planning. Pursuing these goals without having to wait for symptom reduction, or without having to 'prove' their compliance with practitioners' wishes regarding various treatments, inevitably requires services to become more oriented to promoting community inclusion. And, as above, taking charge of their own treatment and recovery planning within a mental health setting may provide valuable learning experiences for people in recovery that can then encourage them to pursue and accept leadership roles in various community organisations and activities, all of which may contribute to their becoming valued citizens of their community.

Finally, it will be equally important to intervene at the practitioner level to ensure that self-determination and community inclusion are encouraged and supported within the mental health system. Previous research has shown that the assumptions described above have led mental health practitioners to stigmatise and limit people in their recovery, and therefore in their efforts towards community inclusion (Brody 2007, Davidson, Stayner and Haglund 1998). In addition to those assumptions described above, such stigma includes beliefs that people with mental illnesses are infantile and in need of care or are responsible for their illness and frequently dangerous. Mental health systems will need to enact policies that indicate zero tolerance for such beliefs and prevent a provider from acting upon those beliefs in a discriminatory fashion.

A related and potentially damaging service provider attitude about people in recovery derives from common misunderstandings and/or misapplications of diagnostic practices. It remains the case that, thirty years after publication of the third edition of the *DSM*, diagnosis still dictates treatment in psychiatry much less than it does in most other medical specialties and, as a result, seldom plays a central role in the care of persons with serious mental illnesses. Instead of taking the time to properly identify, diagnose, and offer education to the person about his or her condition, practitioners are more likely to 'treat the chart' – that is, to utilise diagnostic information to justify the need for treatment and/or establish the person's eligibility for care (Flanagan, Miller and Davidson 2009). As a result, people are denied the opportunity to understand what they are up against or what they can do to enter into and pursue recovery and community life.

Similarly – and again thirty years after publication of the third edition of the *DSM* in which it was made clear that diagnoses refer to psychiatric *conditions* rather than to people – practitioners, researchers, family members, and people with mental illnesses themselves often refer to people by their diagnosis ('schizophrenics', 'borderlines'), suggesting that the disorder is a permanent part of the person and one that defines his or her personhood (Flanagan and Davidson, 2007). While there is considerable longitudinal evidence to the contrary (Davidson, Harding and Spaniol 2005), and while the *DSM* and professional organisations deny that diagnoses are referring to people rather than to conditions, this widespread cultural phenomenon continues to contribute to stigma and discrimination against people with mental illnesses, constituting one of the more formidable barriers to community inclusions.

Additional ways in which practitioners impede the community inclusion of people in recovery may have been implicit in the discussion above, but are nonetheless worth explicating. For example, encouraging a person who has just been diagnosed with a mental illness for the first time to give up his or her hopes and dreams for a contributing life, and to accept instead the life of a mental patient, remains a surprisingly common practice. As a corollary, practitioners also often encourage people with mental illnesses to withdraw from the community and to socialise and enjoy their recreational hobbies in social clubs, day programmes, or other artificial settings that keep them segregated from the community.

For example, rather than encouraging a person in recovery who likes bowling to join a bowling league at the local lanes, practitioners may suggest that the person go bowling with the staff and fellow patients of his or her day care centre. Or rather than encouraging a person in recovery who likes to read to join a book group at the local library, providers may encourage the person to start a book group at his or her local clubhouse day centre – in both cases viewing the person as too 'sick' or 'low functioning' to join in community activities. Similarly, in countries that have relevant legislation to prohibit discrimination in the workplace, practitioners similarly seldom encourage people with mental illnesses to actively seek employment and even more rarely educate people about their right to request the job supports to which they are entitled.

To combat the inertia inherent to these established practices, it will be necessary for mental health systems to implement policies that require practitioners to examine their own potentially damaging beliefs about people in recovery, to make and communicate accurate diagnoses of the conditions people in recovery face, to understand that the diagnosis refers to what the person is up against and not to the person him or herself (Davidson and Strauss 1995), and to offer incentives for practices that enhance, rather than impede, the community inclusion of the people they are entrusted to serve.

Policies focused on the interface between the mental health system and the community

Little thought has been given to the interface between the mental health system and the broader community, beyond the basic assumption that people who need care will be referred to the mental health system and people who benefit from care and recover will rejoin community life. One exception to this customary view has been explored within the last half century, however, largely within Western European countries and beginning, at least by some accounts, with the work of the Basaglias and the Democratic Psychiatry movement they helped to found in Italy in the 1960s. A review of this movement, and the resulting mental health reform in Italy, is beyond the scope of this chapter, and has been described in detail elsewhere (Corbascio and Henry 1994, Crepet 1988, Crepet and Pirella 1985, De Salvia and Williams 1987, Glick 1990, Hanvey 1978, Mangen 1989, Mosher 1983a and 1983b, Ramon 1983). For the purposes of this chapter, we will limit ourselves to four of the key strategies developed by Franco and Franca Basaglia and their colleagues to create more two-way traffic between the mental health system and the community as a step towards closing mental asylums and ensuring 'a life in the community' for all persons with serious mental illnesses – the vision since adopted by the US President's New Freedom Commission on Mental Health (Department of Health and Human Services 2003, Davidson et al. 2010).

Before closing the asylum in Trieste, and as one way of helping the asylum residents to become comfortable being around community people, as well as community people becoming comfortable being around asylum residents, the hospital staff planned public events that would create two-way traffic between the asylum and the community.

In addition to taking patients out of the asylum on community visits, community members were invited onto the grounds of the asylum for a range of publicised cultural, recreational, and social events such as soccer matches, festivals, art exhibits, music concerts, lectures, and other public gatherings. Among this range of activities, those that involved children were especially of interest, both for the salutary effect that the presence of children had for the patients and for the strong challenge this posed to any concerns community members might have had about the potential dangerousness of the patients. Of note, for example, was that a day care centre was established for the children of the staff on the grounds of the asylum and eventually became a valuable asset for the town as a whole. Uninhabited or recently vacated parts of the asylum were put to other uses as well. This became a second key strategy for community inclusion (as well as a step towards honouring the rights of the residents), when the Basaglias terminated the 'work therapy' programme through which residents had cooked meals, did the laundry, helped to take care of the physical facilities, and performed other menial tasks but for which they were paid only in 'tokens' which could be cashed in for cigarettes or other small items. Rather than promoting an artificial 'token economy', a programme was instituted that encouraged residents who were able and interested in working to take on jobs for which they would receive the same level of pay they would have received for the same or similar jobs in the community. This transformation of passive or indentured residents into competitive workers yielded an enormous capacity for employment in a range of industries beyond janitorial and food services, with approximately half of the resident population expressing interest in working. From this modest beginning, and consistent with the principle that citizens have the right to a decent wage for their meaningful labour, the model of social cooperatives was born.

Social cooperatives are industries that employ a mixed workforce, some employees having disabilities and others not. These companies are able to compensate their employees comparable wages to the rest of the business sector, based either on government subsidies used to compensate for reduced productivity or, when possible, on their own self-sustaining productivity. Beginning with their inception in the Trieste asylum, social cooperatives have since become highly visible across the Trieste business sector, at one point numbering forty five different functions. These include cleaning and building maintenance, furniture and design, hotel, cafeteria and restaurant services, agricultural production and gardening, handicraft, carpentry, photo, video and radio production, computer services, theatre, administrative services, and home assistance. It is, in fact, difficult to spend any amount of time in Trieste and not come into contact with a social cooperative in some way. This model has since been replicated in various forms in numerous European countries, Australia and New Zealand. A 1999 survey found that there were about 2,000 social firms in Europe alone, employing approximately 47,000 workers, of whom 40–50 per cent were disabled (Leff and Warner 2006).

A third strategy explored in Trieste was working with organisations and groups that represented other marginalised or disenfranchised people within the community. At the time (the early 1970s), this included the students' movement, the workers' movement, and the feminist movement. Joining forces with such sympathetic movements brought people with mental illnesses into contact with community members, cultivating again two-way traffic between the mental health system and the community. People in recovery discovered that they had much in common, and could socialise with ordinary members of the community, who as a result also found out that people with mental illnesses were in many ways just like them.

A final strategy for promoting inclusion took place at the level of the individual service recipient, and was effective only for one person, one family, or one group at a time. Anticipating perhaps the more recent advances that have been made with supported housing and supported employment, staff worked with each individual to determine the person's interests and needs, and then accompanied the person in his or her efforts to meet his or her needs and pursue his or her interests within the broader community. To do this work, the staff not only had to become adept at recognising and managing the deleterious effects of the illness, but also had to become socially and instrumentally adept at assisting the person in navigating and negotiating the community terrain, whether this be in securing a person's disability pension, resolving conflicts between a person and his or her family, or obtaining the leverage needed to get an unresponsive landlord to repair a leaking sink.

Rather than doing these tasks for the person, which would engender and perpetuate dependence and disability, it was important in such circumstances for the staff's role to be more that of a mediator, who would help community members understand and be responsive to the person with the mental illness while also helping the person with the mental illness to understand how the world works and what it requires from him or her. This kind of *in vivo* mediation, coupled with coaching or mentoring, has since become a core part of the role of the recovery-oriented practitioner (Davidson et al. 2009, Davidson et al. 2006).

Policies focused on the broader community

In terms of the broader community, many of the steps required to foster the inclusion of persons with mental illnesses are similar to, if not the same as, steps that have been taken to foster the inclusion of persons with other illnesses and disabilities, and/or from other historically oppressed minority groups. These steps have included ongoing and aggressive efforts to fight stigma and discrimination in the courts of public opinion and law. Many countries have now passed such legislation, and the EU did in 2001 initiate a policy of social inclusion throughout the European Union (EU COM 2001), which has resulted in a broadening of the attempts of many European countries towards more socially inclusive policy and practice. In America, landmark legislation such as the 1990 Americans with Disabilities Act has had a major impact. Through this law, persons with serious mental illnesses were extended the same rights and protections as persons with physical disabilities, including most fundamentally the right to full inclusion in community life. In addition to these kinds of breakthroughs inspired by the Civil Rights, Feminist, and Gay Rights movements, efforts to promote the community inclusion of persons with mental illnesses can learn from and emulate the relatively recent and successful campaigns for breast cancer awareness and for educational opportunities for children with special needs.

For example, as Jimmie Holland, Chief of Psychiatry of Memorial Sloan-Kettering Cancer Center in the US and a founder of the field of psycho-oncology, points out in her book with Sheldon Lewis (2000), up through the 1960s, cancer carried a powerful stigma for patient and family alike and, indeed, was called the 'Big C' because the word itself was so unacceptable. Holland tells of a watershed event in the 1950s, when two socially prominent New York women, both of whom had radical mastectomies, decided they would try to reach other women to provide a forum in which women could feel free to talk about having breast cancer. They felt that a notice in the *New York Times* was the best way to announce this effort. However, when they called the *Times*, they were told that the paper would not accept a notice using the words 'breast' and 'cancer'. 'Perhaps you could say there will be a meeting about 'diseases of the chest wall,' they were told. Undaunted, the women persisted and their devoted efforts resulted in what is widely known now as Reach to Recovery, a worldwide support programme for women with breast cancer, administered today through the American Cancer Society.

The history of societal attitudes towards children with special needs also parallels in important ways the history of attitudes towards adults with serious mental illnesses. In the past, it was customary for children with physical, medical, and/or emotional challenges to be locked away in distant institutions or at least to be segregated in separate schools or classrooms. They were denied essential opportunities for social and educational development as enjoyed by their more typical peers. It was not until 1975 that the U.S. Congress finally enacted the Education for All Handicapped Children Act (which has since been refined and improved many times over the years and is currently known as the Individuals with Disabilities Education Act). This law, among other things, requires that public school districts throughout the nation place any child with special needs into the regular educational environment unless it is demonstrated through rigorous assessment that education in the regular environment with the use of supplementary aids and services cannot be achieved satisfactorily.

Both of these examples illustrate how increased community awareness brought about through the effort of a group of dedicated people can lead eventually to substantial policy reforms that promote the community inclusion of formerly marginal populations. We suggest that similar steps to those described above for cancer and children with special needs can and should be taken to ensure optimal community inclusion of adults with serious mental illnesses. What remains to be seen are the ways in which current stereotypes of mental illness (for example: risk of dangerousness) may get in the way of such progress, and what creative solutions can be found to overcome these obstacles.

Conclusion

Community inclusion requires the general public to view and treat people with serious mental illnesses first and foremost as citizens rather than as patients, clients, or service users. As a first step in this direction, mental health systems can model acceptance by recognising and valuing the gifts, strengths, skills, talents, interests, and other contributions such people can make to the life of the community. Shortly before his death, Franco Basaglia (1979) asserted that the community itself was enriched through the inclusion of persons with serious mental illnesses and their contributions. As more public figures have disclosed their own histories of mental illness, more and more evidence has accumulated as to the validity and importance of this assertion, paving the way for further and broader inclusion.

Despite these initial promising steps, there remains much work to be done in changing long-standing public perceptions. Therefore we end by invoking the spirit of Philippe Pinel, who, in his 1794 address to the Society for Natural History in Paris, bemoaned the 'many talents lost to Society' due to mental illness and who then suggested that 'great efforts are needed to salvage them!' (Weiner 1992). It is unfortunate that now, over two hundred years later, great efforts continue to be needed.

References

Basaglia, F. (1979). *The Therapeutic Vocation*, in *Scritti* (Torino: Einaudi).
Brody, D. (2007). 'Strategies for Transformation: Identifying, Reducing and Ending Discrimination and Stigma in Mental Health and Primary Care Settings', *Improving Provider Attitudes, Behaviors and Practices Toward People with Mental Illness. Teleconference Sponsored by the SAMHSA Resource Center to Address Discrimination and Stigma*, November 2009.
Corbascio, G. and Henry, P. (1994). 'How Can Psychiatry Survive without Psychiatric Hospitals? The Italian Experience', *International Journal of Social Psychiatry*, XL, 269–75.
Crepet, P. (1988). 'The Italian Mental Health Reform Nine Years On', *Acta Psychiatrica Scandinavica*, LXXVII, 5–23.
Crepet, P. and Pirella, A. (1985). 'The Transformation of Psychiatric Care in Italy: Methodological Premises, Current Status and Future Prospects', *International Journal of Mental Health*, XIV, 55–73.
Davidson, L. (1997). 'Vulnérabilité et destin dans la schizophrénie: Prêter l'oreille á la voix de la personne' [Vulnerability and Destiny in Schizophrenia: Hearkening to the Voice of the Person], *L'évolution psychiatrique*, LXII, 263–84.
Davidson, L., Harding, C. M. and Spaniol, L. (2005). *Recovery from Severe Mental Illnesses: Research Evidence and Implications for Practice*, vol. 1 (Boston, MA: Center for Psychiatric Rehabilitation of Boston University).
Davidson, L., Mezzina, R., Rowe, M. and Thompson, K. (2010) 'A Life in the Community, Italian Mental Health Reform and Recovery', *Journal of Mental Health*, 19(5), 436–43.
Davidson, L. and Roe, D. (2007). 'Recovery from versus Recovery in Serious Mental Illness: One Strategy for Lessening Confusion Plaguing Recovery', *Journal of Mental Health*, XVI(4), 1–12.
Davidson, L., Stayner, D. and Haglund, K. E. (1998). 'Phenomenological Perspectives on the Social Functioning of People with Schizophrenia', in K. T. Mueser and N. Tarrier (eds). *Handbook of Social Functioning in Schizophrenia* (Boston: Allyn and Bacon), 97–120.
Davidson, L. and Strauss, J. S. (1995). 'Beyond the Biopsychosocial Model: Integrating Disorder, Health and Recovery', *Psychiatry: Interpersonal and Biological Processes*, LVIII, 44–55.
Davidson, L., Tondora, J., O'Connell, M. J., Lawless, M. S. and Rowe, M. (2009). *A Practical Guide to Recovery-Oriented Practice: Tools for Transforming Mental Health Care* (New York: Oxford University Press).
Davidson, L., Tondora, J. S., Staeheli, M. R., O'Connell, M. J., Frey, J. and Chinman, M. J. (2006). 'Recovery Guides: An Emerging Model of Community-Based

Care for Adults with Psychiatric Disabilities', in A. Lightburn and P. Sessions (eds). *Community-Based Clinical Practice* (London: Oxford University Press), 476–501.

Department of Health and Human Services (2003). *Achieving the Promise: Transforming Mental Health Care in America* (Rockville, MD: Substance Abuse and Mental Health Services Administration).

De Salvia, D. and Williams, P. (1987). 'The Italian Experience and its Implications', *Psychological Medicine*, XVII, 283–9.

EU COM (2001) 'Joint Report on Social Inclusion'. Brussels: Commission of the European Communities.

Fitch, C., Daw, R., Balmer, N., Gray, K. and Skipper, M. (2008). *Fair Deal for Mental Health: Our Manifesto for a 3-Year Campaign Dedicated to Tackling Inequality in Mental Healthcare* (London, England: Royal College of Psychiatrists).

Flanagan, E. H. and Davidson, L. (2007). '"Schizophrenics", "Borderlines", and the Lingering Legacy of "Misplaced Concreteness": The Persistent Misconception that the DSM Classifies People Instead of Disorders', *Psychiatry: Interpersonal and Biological Processes*, LXX(2), 100–12.

Flanagan, E. H., Miller, R. and Davidson, L. (2009). '"Unfortunately We Treat the Chart": Sources of Stigma in Mental Health Settings", *Psychiatric Quarterly*, LXXX(1), 55–64.

Glick, I. D. (1990). 'Improving Treatment for the Severely Mentally Ill: Implications of the Decade-Long Italian Psychiatric Reform', *Psychiatry*, LIII, 316–23.

Hanvey, C. (1978). 'Italy and the Rise of Democratic Psychiatry', *Community Care*, XXV, 22–4.

Holland, J. and Lewis, S. (2000). *The Human Side of Cancer* (New York: Harper Collins).

Leff, J. and Warner, R. (2006). *Social Inclusion of People with Mental Illness* (Cambridge, UK, Cambridge University Press), 139.

Mangen, S. P. (1989). 'The Politics of Reform: Origins and Enactment of the Italian Experience', *International Journal of Social Psychiatry*, XXXV, 7–19.

Mosher, L. R. (1983a). 'Radical Deinstitutionalization: The Italian Experience', *International Journal of Mental Health*, XI, 129–36.

Mosher, L. R. (1983b). 'Recent Developments in the Care, Treatment, and Rehabilitation of the Chronic Mentally Ill in Italy', *Hospital and Community Psychiatry*, XXXIV, 947–50.

Ramon, S. (1983). 'Psichiatria Democratica: A Case Study of an Italian Community Mental Health Service', *International Journal of Health Services*, XIII(2), 307–24.

Tondora, J., Pocklington, S., Gorges, A., Osher, D. and Davidson, L. (2005). *Implementation of Person-Centered Care and Planning. From Policy to Practice to Evaluation* (Washington D.C.: Substance Abuse and Mental Health Services Administration).

Weiner, D. B. (1992). 'Pinel's "Memoir on Madness" of December 11, 1794: A Fundamental Text of Modern Psychiatry', *American Journal of Psychiatry*, CXLIX, 725–32.

7
Employment and Social Inclusion: Implementing the Model and Facing the Reality

Justine Schneider

Background

Employment is recognised by professionals and service users as a key element in facilitating both social inclusion and recovery for people with the lived experience of mental ill health. Over half a million people of working age in the UK have a mental health-related disability. Although severe mental illness such as schizophrenia or bipolar disorder affects a minority – less than two per cent of the general population – having such a problem makes it much more likely that an adult of working age with this disability is unemployed than people with other disabilities: 18 per cent in work compared to 48 per cent in one recent study (Smith and Twomey 2002). It is not known to what extent the discrepancy between employment rates of people disabled by mental health problems and people with other disabilities is due to stigma, to low expectations on the part of mental health services or to lack of aspirations on the part of service users. It is clear, however, that substitutes for paid employment are not acceptable outcomes for most mental health service users: education, volunteering and work experience may have a part to play in recovery, but they would not be regarded as definitive alternatives to paid work by anyone in pursuit of a real job (ODPM 2004). For adults of working age in our society, having paid employment is an incomparable source of identity, social status, economic independence and purpose in life.

The current economic crisis is an inescapable factor in discussions about work for people with disabilities in many European countries. Several reasons combine to make it a minor consideration. Firstly, it can be argued that there is a need to plan for the future and the anticipated improvement in the economy. Secondly, on the principle of equal opportunity, it can be argued that people facing the greatest disadvantage should get the most help into work, as a matter of justice. Finally, it is sometimes observed that the entry level and part-time jobs, which people with mental health problems often use as their stepping-stones into the labour market, may be affected less than other types of employment in a recession.

Evidence for individual placement and support (IPS)

Supported employment, broadly defined, has been provided for people with disabilities in the UK for many years, both through government programmes promoting welfare to work, and through public, voluntary and private sector providers (Wistow and Schneider 2007). Traditionally, like other people who have severe disabilities or long-term health conditions, people with long-term or severe mental health problems rarely make the transition from inactivity into employment; often they get stuck in a cycle of endless training and job preparation. To overcome this, an approach to employment support known as Individual Placement and Support (IPS) has been developed and tested extensively and is today recognised in practice guidelines and in policy recommendations as an effective means to help individuals with severe mental health problems who wish to work (DOH 2006, Perkins et al. 2009).

A meta-analysis of 11 largely US randomised controlled studies of IPS found an overall employment rate of 61 per cent compared to 23 per cent for controls (Bond, Drake and Becker 2008). These studies include a European trial, EQOLISE (Burns et al. 2007), which makes an important contribution to the IPS literature because, as the authors state: 'Europe differs greatly from the USA in both its employment practices (varying amounts of employment protection compared with a hire and fire culture in the USA) and in having more generous welfare systems. Such systems might generate a benefit trap, in which there could be perceived or real financial disincentives to returning to work – for example, loss of housing benefits or high disability payments' (p. 1146). In keeping with the US studies, EQOLISE took at least one day in paid employment as its main outcome. By this criterion, IPS was more effective, with 55% gaining work compared to 28 per cent of people in non-IPS vocational services. Moreover, IPS beneficiaries worked on average twice as much (214 days) as controls (108 days). Effectiveness varied between countries, however; the significant difference favouring IPS were observed in London (England), Rimini (Italy), Zurich (Switzerland) and Sofia (Bulgaria), but not in Ulm (Germany), where a high number of people in the control group got work, nor in Gronigen (Netherlands). The perceived disincentive to work due to reductions in benefits entitlements, and the buoyancy of the local labour markets were identified by Burns et al. (2007) as factors affecting their results. Contrary to expectations, a UK study by Howard et al. (2010) failed to produce a significant difference, probably because it was not sufficiently intensive, described by Latimer (2010) as an effective intervention delivered at a sub-therapeutic dose.

Overall, it is fair to infer from the evidence that the employment outcomes for IPS are broadly twice as good as for the non-IPS employment support services studied. All vocational services are focussed on paid work as a key outcome: what then are the distinctive features of IPS? The U.S. Substance Abuse and Mental Health Services Administration describes seven principles: competitive employment, zero exclusion, rapid placement and support, individualised support tailored to personal preferences, open-ended access to IPS expertise, integration with clinical services, and welfare benefits counselling (SAMHSA 2009).

First, the emphasis on competitive employment means that alternatives such as training, sheltered work or lengthy job preparation are not considered in IPS. By comparison, alternative services may endorse education or voluntary work as outcomes. The take-home message of IPS is 'place-train instead of train-place'; it rejects drawn-out preparations for work, along with sheltered work environments and other ways of organising employment where people with mental health problems are segregated from the general workforce. This feature may demand a cultural change for service providers and users accustomed to the train-place philosophy. Indeed, some carers and even some clinicians may find that the place-train approach confronts them with a loss of control over the service user which they deem unacceptably risky. There is no objective evidence that IPS increases risks to its users; in the EQOLISE study, for example, IPS users were less, not more likely to be readmitted to hospital than users of traditional vocational support (Burns et al. 2007).

Second, the philosophy underpinning IPS is to assume that no person is excluded from work by their diagnosis alone ('zero exclusion'). Zero exclusion alarms some people because it is a radical concept: no person is deemed to be unable to work. This does not mean that all people have an equal likelihood of working. People with severe mental health problems face particular barriers in relation to their specific impairments and for some people these present severe challenges to employment (McGurk and Mueser 2004). Some people's lives are further complicated by welfare benefits status, substance use, poor social skills or a history of violent behaviour. These issues cannot be ignored, but neither do they determine employability; they are given due consideration in the assessment and placement of individuals. Zero exclusion means that an employment service offers equal access to all, despite work history, symptoms or diagnosis. The zero exclusion approach fosters a positive attitude on the part of all concerned, and this optimism about employment potential should pervade the organisations involved, so that their policies and practices as well as their personnel actively challenge the prejudice that people with mental health problems are not employable.

Other key principles of IPS state that job search should start soon after a person decides to seek employment (normally within one month), and should be driven by a person's preference and choice. If new skills are needed, they should ideally be acquired on the job, through job-coaching or using the training opportunities available from the employer. Employment specialists work closely with the service user and the employer to identify and negotiate any disability-related workplace adjustments required.

An important requirement of IPS is that employment specialists and clinical teams are integrated and co-located, so that employment support and clinical care may be closely co-ordinated. This represents the biggest adaptation for mental health services. Where it is achieved, it seems to generate a virtuous circle of communication and collaboration between employment specialists and clinical staff, which serves to educate each group about the other's domain of expertise, to the benefit of service users (Latimer 2010).

Furthermore, support is not time-limited and can be accessed by the employer as well as the employee, provided the employee has chosen to disclose the purpose of the service to their employer. Finally and fundamentally, welfare benefits counselling is part of the service; this includes ensuring that hours of employment and pay are coordinated with benefit plans developed with expert advisers. Although there are real disincentives to paid work in some social security systems, in the UK these have been reduced over time. Nonetheless staff and user perceptions of the 'benefits trap' have not necessarily kept pace with these changes, so up-to-date expert assessment is essential.

The IPS fidelity scale

As shown earlier, the evidence of effectiveness for IPS is strong. Moreover, the technical requirements are clear and explicit. In addition to the functional aspects of IPS outlined above, there are a number of organisational criteria used to establish the 'fidelity' of an IPS service. These include caseload size, the amount of time employment specialists spend offering support (as compared to other job roles), their level of specialisation in the role, their integration with mental health providers, their links with external rehabilitation services, and the way the vocational service is structured within the larger mental health agency (Supported Employment Fidelity Scale, 2008). These 'fidelity criteria' may be used to judge the level of development of IPS in a mental health context. For example:

- each Supported employment (SE) specialist should be working with no more than 20 individuals,
- the SE specialists are fully integrated with the mental health team
- the SE unit is led by an SE team leader.

There is evidence linking some of these fidelity criteria to outcomes (Bond 2004). Their main application is to monitor and evaluate service adherence and determine to what degree a given employment support service achieves the IPS standard approach to supported employment by scoring the results on a scale rated 'high', 'fair', 'low' and 'no' fidelity.

From theory to practice

In mental health care, as in any service sector, knowing what works and actually doing it are sometimes difficult to reconcile. Putting new approaches into practice can be made more difficult by entrenched attitudes, organisational inertia and competing priorities, notwithstanding resource limitations. Including people with disabilities in the workforce is a challenge. Including people with severe mental illness such as schizophrenia or bipolar disorder may seem even more difficult, but it has been achieved in many countries using a systematic approach.

Experience with implementing IPS

Becker et al. (1998), after implementing IPS in several community mental health services in the US, identified five key issues around implementation: leadership, organisational structure, training, finance and time frames. First, leaders function as role models and can develop a culture of change through good communication and feedback. In the US, it emerged that most leaders were the executive directors who managed key staff members and who could empower them to overcome barriers of change; but of course 'leadership' can come from any quarter, including service users.

Second, the integration of rehabilitation services and mental health treatments is crucial. This implies restructuring community mental health teams and (at least) weekly meetings for the new, integrated teams. Third, all staff members need a clear understanding of the IPS model, including the principles, goals and implementation criteria. Therefore it is important that expert training for IPS is provided to all, with ongoing supervision in order to reinforce this. Fourth, mental health services need resources to replace usual services with a new approach; this presents a familiar challenge of 'double-funding' of parallel services through a period of transition. Becker et al. (1998) noted that, in the US context, it takes up to a year to implement IPS: this includes restructuring services, helping staff to train and removing barriers or resistance to change. A realistic timescale is helpful to manage expectations.

Building on the work of Becker and his colleagues, and still in the US context, Marshall et al. (2008) identified three keys to success in implementation. First, having a strong leader who takes a hands-on approach, with freedom to hire and fire employment specialists, who gives direct feedback on performance and makes clear what is expected in terms of the employment specialists' day-to-day work. Second, it seems important for the employment specialists to have previous experience of clinical, mental health services. An understanding of the experience of mental illness equips employment specialists to work more effectively with the client group. Indeed, they are more confident in marketing the skills of potential employees and representing their interests with employers if they have a clinical background. Thirdly, staff attitudes appear to be critical. Clearly, they need to be in favour of employment as an outcome for service users, so a service ethos that promotes recovery and social inclusion is desirable, although Marshall et al. (2008) observed that staff behaviour was not always consistent with 'zero exclusion' as defined earlier in this chapter. The factors emphasised by the latter authors may be summarised as leadership, expert knowledge about the field on the part of employment support providers, and commitment on the part of mental health staff.

Rinaldi, Miller and Perkins (2010) draw on experience of introducing IPS into two UK mental health services to elaborate on the particular implementation issues they encountered, since 'there are cultural differences between countries, along with considerable differences between health, social care, employment and welfare systems, which demand consideration of how IPS can be implemented within different countries and contexts' (p. 165). They highlight three stages of IPS implementation: adoption in principle, early implementation and persistence of implementation. The first concerns changing attitudes and expectations;

leadership and senior management support are essential at this stage. The second stage is described in terms of bringing about a paradigm shift in mental health services, fostering familiarity with IPS practice and evidence, measuring early outcomes, and feeding them back, with incremental growth in service provision. Persistence or mainstreaming has led to the development of cross-organisational partnerships, underpinned by the application of the IPS Fidelity Scale, and going on to offer career development opportunities for people in work.

Implementation of IPS in Nottingham: a practice example

In this section, the implementation of IPS in Nottingham during its first year of operation is described. The local policy context for implementation of IPS in Nottingham was favourable: for more than a decade, UK policy has been geared towards encouraging people into work. Consequently, all disabled people, including those with mental health problems, face a benefits environment that is now structured to reward efforts made towards gaining employment. This policy environment has become even stricter in this regard with for example the national introduction of the Employment and Support Allowance in 2008 – a new and greatly simplified benefits regime oriented towards return to work. The policy environment is therefore conducive to employment initiatives targeted at people with mental health problems. Yet it is not uncontested. For instance, Rinaldi, Miller and Perkins (2010) identify four impediments: fear and prejudice on the part of the people concerned; a culture of low expectations in relation to people with mental health difficulties; an ingrained bias towards 'train-place' approaches to rehabilitation despite evidence to the contrary; and the impact of the global recession.

There was also a fairly compelling case for change. Nottingham is right in the centre of England, it has an urban population approaching 300,000 inhabitants and it has a largely post-industrial economy. Between 1956 and 1961, Mapperley Hospital in Nottingham, together with Netherne to the south of London and Severalls on the outskirts of Colchester, participated in the seminal 'three hospitals' study reported in *Schizophrenia and Social Care* (Brown, Bone, Dalison and Wing 1966), a landmark in social psychiatric research. Brown and colleagues followed 339 people admitted to these hospitals with a diagnosis of schizophrenia. At that time, researchers were disappointed that 'only' 40% were working, a level of employment that would be a distant hope today. An internal audit of the service in question in 2008 showed that only 14 per cent of people on the secondary care teams' caseloads were in any form of work, paid or unpaid. Of course, the workforce has changed a lot in the past 50 years, with fewer unskilled or semi-skilled factory jobs now than before. Major employers used to be a bicycle maker and a cigarette manufacturer; now a university stands on the same site. The service industries that have replaced factories do not need large numbers of unskilled workers. A person whose illness inter-rupts their education puts them at a disadvantage in the labour market. In addition, the threshold for admission to high levels of support from mental health services has risen, more people are treated in primary care and those seen by community mental health teams may be as severely disabled as the people who were hospitalised 50 years ago.

Tailoring the service

In 2009, when the Nottingham IPS development project began, there was an established employment support service in the Nottingham mental health service, employing three part-time staff, although it was not co-located with clinical teams. Most rehabilitation resources were invested in specialist centres staffed mainly by occupational therapists focused on skills acquisition and confidence building, although this resource (approximately 30 staff) was small in relation to the service-user population of more than 2,000. There was a history of embattle-ment: any rumour of change was met with organised resistance on the part of people who felt threatened by this, whether they were staff, service users, their carers or even Members of Parliament. Winning over public opinion was therefore an important objective. To promote consistency of practice and launch the new IPS service, both existing and new employment support staff were re-branded as a single service (*Bridgebuilders*) and marketed to potential users including employers, a departure from previous practice which had been focused exclusively on the needs of service users with mental health problems.

Training

In keeping with implementation recommendations, (Becker et al. 1998) training Trust staff was given high priority and specialist training in IPS was delivered by outside experts to the Trust's vocational rehabilitation service staff and to employment specialists. The staff who had been trained were supported to practice in new ways, with occupational therapists, occupational therapy technical instructors and others in the social inclusion and vocational rehabilitation service becoming potential agents for change in implementing the new service. Yet they are a minority of the staff complement and, as we shall see below, they found themselves – and this is still the case today – up against organisational changes that sometimes appear to be in contradiction with certain of the principles of IPS.

Leadership and expert knowledge

The active support of key directors and senior professionals is seen by Rinaldi, Miller and Perkins (2010) as a necessary condition of organisational change, as is the commitment of the managers who determine what happens in community mental health teams; but, as these authors point out, 'the most powerful evidence is when front-line mental health professionals can see service users gaining employment with their own eyes' (p. 168).

Essential to the Nottingham initiative was the recruitment of an 'IPS Development Manager', designed to facilitate the new service. This was a completely new post, which meant gaining approval for the job description before it could be advertised. It was essentially a specialised change management role, and the recruitment to the post of an experienced employment support manager from outside the NHS brought the expert knowledge about IPS that was known to be an essential requirement. With a time-limited contract and conscious of the need to develop local expertise and 'ownership' of IPS, the Development Manager worked strategically to establish familiarity with local policies, build and inform networks of key staff by means of targeted marketing and communications and embed the seven principles of IPS in the Trust's systems of management and appraisal. Supported by the Centre for Mental Health (formerly the Sainsbury Centre for Mental Health) through its Centres of Excellence in the IPS national programme, he received high-level mentorship and training from the team at Dartmouth, New Hampshire in the US, where IPS was first codified and disseminated (SAMHSA, 2009).

The Development Manager tackled the immediate organisational issues by undertaking a fidelity review of existing services and developing an IPS implementation plan which was agreed and monitored by the IPS steering group. Key elements of the plan included: co-location of employment specialists with mental health teams, reliable capture of output data for performance management purposes and clear definition of service-level objectives.

Facilitation

Facilitation of change was deliberately addressed in every project within CLAHRC-NDL (Collaboration for Leadership in Applied Health Research and Care - Nottinghamshire, Derbyshire and Lincolnshire) through the adoption of a 'Diffusion Fellow' model. Diffusion Fellows are middle to senior managers from the local health provider, seconded by their employer for one day per week to work with a research team. In this project, a senior physiotherapist agreed to participate as a champion for IPS in the Trust, by advising the project on Trust practices and occasionally contacting colleagues to unblock administrative bottlenecks. As a person who will hopefully remain in the Trust when the project has ended, the Diffusion Fellow carries forward the ethos of IPS and is instrumental in embedding it in the developing organisation.

Monitoring of the Nottingham implementation

Monitoring and feedback were obtained through an independent fidelity review conducted after three months of operation. It highlighted several shortfalls in implementation, three of which are outlined here. Preliminary evaluations revealed low caseload turnover due in part to old clients remaining on the caseload – up to 4 years. We found that some process records were not being completed, so there was no evidence of whether or how certain formal assessments were made. This revealed an issue around management capacity. Supervision of the specialists had been replaced largely by 'peer support' – weekly meetings but with little or no quality monitoring. A survey of care co-ordinators showed that employment specialists were not spending much time in the team, and that mental health staff were unclear about the IPS service. It was even alleged that some referrals had been rejected, in contravention of the principle of zero exclusion. A fidelity review three months into the service showed that it was not up to IPS standard. One year on, fidelity was independently rated as 'good'.

Three considerations are relevant to wider IPS implementation. First, the major organisational requirement, insertion of employment staff in community mental health teams, met delays of several months due to a wholesale reconfiguration of mental health teams in the city. Second, the manager of the employment specialists was not entirely dedicated to IPS. According to IPS Fidelity criteria, one full time supervisor should manage no more than ten employment specialists. However, the manager in question was responsible for more than 30 'vocational' staff, and only two of them were employment specialists following the IPS model. This limits severely the amount of hands-on support and modelling which the supervisor could do. A third issue, not previously identified, concerns the size of the mental health team into which the employment specialists were linked. Driven by the need to make 'efficiency savings', the team to which the employment specialists are attached was amalgamated with several others which formerly operated in distinct geographical sectors. It numbers 70 care co-ordinators and allied staff, making the employment specialist resource sorely inadequate and posing challenges to communication and co-ordination about individual service users.

The action plan to resolve these challenges included: full co-location of employment specialists with the mental health service; the IPS Development Manager leading weekly meetings with the employment specialists using management by objectives; renewed publicity with expert advice on marketing; open meetings for service users to stimulate interest in IPS; extending the service to people who currently get less psychiatric intervention; and another fidelity review after 3 months.

With time-limited funding, there is a risk that the problems cannot be resolved in time to achieve full-fidelity IPS and generate the desired outcomes. At worst, we may learn from the process and disseminate this learning for others to avoid the pitfalls.

Looking to the future and how to make IPS sustainable in the UK, one important area to emphasise appears to be the cost-effectiveness of employment support. Indeed, cuts in UK public sector funding affect both the NHS and local authority social care, as well as the voluntary sector which depends on grants from these two bodies. Planning for austerity, many services are retracting to their statutory minimum. No commitment to service provision is planned except to those activities that are required by law. This implies that employment support needs to be recognised as an essential part of mental health care if IPS in its effective, co-located form is to survive. The essential part played by IPS in the widely-advocated recovery approach to mental health care needs to be emphasised: an indicator of recovery is employment. In addition, it is of key importance to assemble evidence for the savings to mental health services that can reasonably be gained from an effective employment support service. In the US, Bush et al. (2009) conducted a review of the service use impact of employment and concluded that 'Highly significant reductions in service use were associated with steady employment' (p. 1024). Hence, it is reasonable to expect that longer-term follow-ups of people receiving employment support will demonstrate cumulative savings to service providers and increased tax revenue from effective employment support along IPS lines.

In conclusion, the context for the adoption of IPS in Nottingham is in many ways favourable, and consistent with implementation science theory as well as with specific recommendations for IPS implementers. The local context benefits from expert leadership, training, active change management and forward planning. Despite these strengths, several months after the launch of the service and two years into the IPS implementation project, the service did not yet fully meet internationally recognised fidelity criteria. While specific remedies were evident, structural problems arising from service reorganisation remained, due in part to the UK's economic recession, which was deeper than in a number of other European countries. A concerted effort to amass reliable evidence of the longer-term cost-effectiveness of employment support should help to secure the future of this evidence-based approach to mental health care.

References

Becker, D. R., Torrey, W. C., Toscano, R., Wyzik, P. F. and Fox, T. S. (1998). 'Building Recovery- Oriented Services: Lessons Learned from Implementing Individual Placement and Support (IPS) in Community Mental Health Centres', *Psychiatric Rehabilitation Journal*, XXII, 51–4.

Bond, G. R. (2004). 'Supported Employment: Evidence for an Evidence-Based Practice', *Psychiatric Rehabilitation Journal*, XXVII, 345–59.

Bond, G. R., Drake, R. E. and Becker, D. R. (2008). 'An Update on Randomized Controlled Trials of Evidence-Based Supported Employment', *Psychiatric Rehabilitation Journal*, XXXI, 280–90.

Brown, G. W., Bone, M., Dalison, B. and Wing, J. K. (1966). *Schizophrenia and Social Care: A Comparative Follow-up of 339 Schizophrenic Patients* (London: Oxford University Press), Maudsley Monograph No. 17.

Burns, T., Catty, J., Becker, T., Drake, R. E., Fioritti, A., Knapp, M. et al. (2007). 'The Effectiveness of Supported Employment for People with Severe Mental Illness: A Randomised Controlled Trial', *Lancet*, CCCLXX, 1146–52.

Bush, P. W., Drake, R. E., Haiyi, X., McHugo, G. J. and Haslett, W. R. (2009). 'The Long-Term Impact of Employment on Mental Health Service Use and Costs for Persons with Severe Mental Illness', *Psychiatric Services*, LX, 1024–31.

Department of Health (DOH), Department for Work and Pensions (2006). *Vocational Services for People with Severe Mental Health Problems: Commissioning Guidance* (London: Department of Health).

Howard, L. M., Heslin, M., Leese, M., McCrone, P., Rice, C., Jarrett, M. et al. (2010). 'Supported Employment: Randomised Controlled Trial', *Br J Psychiatry*, CXCVI, 404–11.

Latimer, E. (2010). 'An Effective Intervention Delivered at Sub-Therapeutic Dose becomes an Ineffective Intervention, Editorial, *The British Journal of Psychiatry*, CXCVI, 341–2.

Marshall, T., Rapp, C. A., Becker, D. R., Bond, G. R. (2008). 'Key Factors for Implementing Supported Employment', *Psychiatric Services*, LIX, 886–92.

McGurk, S. and Mueser, K. (2004). 'Cognitive Functioning, Symptoms and Work in Supported Employment: A Review and Heuristic Model', *Schizophrenia Research*, LXX, 147–74. doi: 10.1016/j.schres.2004.01.009.

ODPM (Office of the Deputy Prime Minister) (2004). *Social Exclusion Unit Report: Mental Health and Social Exclusion* (London: ODPM).

Perkins, R. (2009). *Realizing Ambitions: Better Employment Support for People with Mental Health Problems* (London: Department of Work and Pensions).

Rinaldi, M., Miller, L. and Perkins, R. (2010). 'Implementing the Individual Placement and Support (IPS) Approach for People with Mental Health Conditions in England', *International Review of Psychiatry*, XXII, 163–72.

Smith, A. and Twomey, B. (2002) (Labour Market Division, Office of National Statistics Labour Market). *Experiences of People with Disabilities: An Examination of the Characteristics of People with Disabilities and How They Fare in the Labour Market Using Up-to-Date Analysis from the Labour Force Survey*. http://www.social-firms.co.uk/system/files/Labour%20market%20experiences%20of%20people%20with%20disabilities,%20August%202002.pdf, date accessed 29 June 2011.

Substance Abuse and Mental Health Services Administration (SAMHSA) (2009). *Supported Employment: Getting Started with Evidence-Based Practices*. DHHS Pub. No. SMA-08-4364, (Rockville, MD: Center for Mental Health Services, Substance Abuse and Mental Health Services Administration, U.S. Department of Health and Human Services). http://www.parecovery.org/documents/AHCI_Supported_Employment_071009.pdf, date accessed 2 May 2011.

Supported Employment Fidelity Scale (2008). http://www.ohiosamiccoe.cwru.edu/library/media/sefidelityscale.pdf, date accessed 3 December 2010.

Wistow, R. and Schneider, J. (2007). 'Supported Employment Agencies in the UK: Current Operation and Future Development Needs', *Health & Social Care in the Community*, XV, 128–35.

8
Overcoming Barriers to Empowerment

Tim Greacen and Emmanuelle Jouet

The aim of this chapter is to describe how institutions working in the area of mental health identify, handle and overcome obstacles to user empowerment through access to lifelong learning and employment. Although individual psychological and psychosocial problems are traditionally identified as the major problem area, macrosocial and institutional problems, ranging from high local unemployment rates through to institutional inertia are also significant. The chapter reviews the scientific literature on this question and describes how partners in the EMILIA project shared information across all eight European sites to develop two implementation tools: the Pathways Readiness Evaluation Tool (PRET), an aid for users to develop individual lifelong learning and employment projects, and the Service and Institution Readiness Checklist (SIRC), designed to assist agencies and organisations to overcome barriers to empowerment.

Context

In March 2000, the Lisbon Summit of the European Council set an ambitious policy for lifelong learning with the explicit objective of making the European Union the 'the most competitive and dynamic knowledge-based economy in the world capable of sustainable economic growth with more and better jobs and greater social cohesion' by 2010 (Council of the European Union 2000). Economic growth through lifelong learning, employment and social inclusion were the foundations of Union policy.

However, throughout the ten years that followed, the difficulties of applying the Lisbon strategy to socially excluded groups such as people with serious and enduring mental illness rapidly became obvious (Ogunleye 2009). Indeed, the rates of unemployment for people diagnosed with severe mental illness throughout Europe are high. European countries that have collected data on this question report employment rates from 12–25 per cent (Kilian and Becker 2007, Linhorst 2006). People with mental health problems have a significantly lower chance of obtaining employment compared to individuals with other disabilities (Berthoud 2006, Kilian and Becker 2007) or compared to the general population of comparable age (Marwaha and Johnson 2004; Smith and Twomey 2002). They are also more likely to be in unskilled employment rather than having jobs corresponding to their potential. Young people with severe mental illness often experience long-term unemployment problems following interruptions to secondary and post-secondary education (Mowbray, Collins and Bybee 1999).

The success of the supported employment (SE) model for the social inclusion of individuals with other disabilities (Gilson 1998, Wehman and Revell 2005) has led to its adaptation for people with serious ongoing mental illness, with considerably improved outcomes in terms of obtaining and maintaining employment compared to traditional approaches using sheltered workshops or rehabilitation training, both in the US (Bond et al. 2008) and in Europe (Burns et al. 2007, 2008). With regard to accessing lifelong learning, a Supported Education model has grown up parallel to the SE model. Supported Education is a recovery-oriented practice that generally targets post-secondary or vocational education with continuing on-campus or off-campus support for people with serious mental illness who wish to return to school or university to complete their educational goals. Research has shown benefits in terms of educational attainment and competitive employment (Mowbray, Collins and Bybee 1999, Mowbray et al. 2005), number of days hospitalised (Insenwater et al. 2002) as well as self-esteem, empowerment and user satisfaction (Danley 1997, Collins, Bybee and Mowbray 1998).

The SE model is being increasingly recommended across Europe (Pallisera, Vila and Valls 2003). However, although more successful than traditional approaches, even these supported programmes can founder if they are not structurally integrated into existing mental health services or if in the presence of financial disincentives with regard to social benefits (Howard et al. 2010). Indeed, rigorous Individual Placement and Support (IPS) programmes manage to obtain sustained employment only for a part of the total population of people with serious mental illness (Drake et al. 1996a). For people who do not work or for whom these supported programmes do not work, other measures will be necessary to promote social inclusion (Howard et al. 2010).

Obstacles and facilitators to accessing training and employment for this population can be encountered from individual level through to institutional and macrosocial levels.

Obstacles and facilitators at the individual level

Although early reviews of the SE literature underline how little individual client factors such as diagnosis, symptoms, age, gender, disability status, prior hospitalisation, education and co-occurring substance abuse predict employment outcomes (Bond et al. 2001), more recent studies are less affirmative. Clients with less severe thought disorder symptoms are more likely to obtain competitive employment (Campbell et al. 2010). Individuals with higher levels of cognitive impairment may require more vocational support, with closer monitoring and more frequent prompts (McGurk et al. 2003, Liberman 2008). Recent hospitalisation is associated with less successful outcomes both in the US (Razzano et al. 2005) and in Europe (Burns et al. 2009). Similarly, the presence of psychiatric symptoms is associated with less successful outcomes (Burns et al. 2009) and this has been found to be true for both negative (Razzano et al. 2005) or positive (McGurk et al. 2003) symptoms. Managing one's symptoms sufficiently to be able to do the job at the right time within a workplace context and developing appropriate coping skills play a large role in finding and maintaining work (Becker et al. 2007, Linhorst 2006). Better global functioning (Burns et al. 2009) and self-rated functioning (Razzano et al. 2005) at baseline are predictors of employment outcomes. Social skills are essential for enduring employment (Liberman 2008) and better social skills at baseline predict working at 18 months (Burns et al. 2009). Having a good level of social adjustment also often means having a stronger social network and therefore easier access to jobs (Collins, Mowbray and Bybee 2000). IPS programmes with additional work-related social skills training (Tsang et al. 2008) or cognitive training (McGurk et al. 2007) obtain higher employment rates and longer job tenure than IPS without this additional training.

The individual's work and training experience are major factors predicting positive outcomes. Educational attainment is associated with greater employment rates for individuals with severe mental illness (Australian Bureau of Statistics 2008, Waghorn, Chant and Whiteford 2003). Similarly, having worked prior to illness leads to better chances for working once the illness has declared itself (Gioia 2005). In a review of four randomized control IPS studies, work history was the only systematic predictor for job acquisition, with people who had been out of work longer being less likely to get a job (Schneider et al. 2009), a result recently confirmed in a multisite European IPS project (Catty et al. 2008). Being in education or work at baseline is a significant factor in predicting a positive outcome at follow-up (Collins, Mowbray and Bybee 2000). Finding work that matches the candidate's job preferences is associated with increased job tenure and satisfaction (Mueser, Becker and Wolfe 2001), with motivational interviewing increasingly being recommended to help people with severe mental illness into work (Drake and Bond 2008, Howard et al. 2010). Participants often prefer part-time work, perceived as being less demanding and less likely to trigger mental health problems (McGurk et al. 2003). Identifying and responding to individual training and educational needs enable clients to move to better jobs and have a more satisfying career (Baron and Salzer 2000, Linhorst 2006), their career aspirations often having been held in check by interrupted secondary or post-secondary education (Kirsner 2009).

In summary, although early studies refuted the idea that individual factors such as diagnosis, cognitive impairment, social skills or work history influence access to work in any major way, more recent research underlines the importance of taking them into account, particularly if job tenure and satisfaction are integrated into programme objectives.

Obstacles and facilitators at the institutional level

Having fewer met social needs is associated with more successful employment outcomes (Catty et al. 2008). The negative impact of having benefits is well documented in the US (Kanter 2008, Campbell 2010) and in Europe (Pallisera, Vila and Valls 2003), with people without disabilities pensions generally faring better in terms of accessing and maintaining work integration than people on pensions (Bond et al. 2007). Van Erp et al. (2007), in a multi-site study in the Netherlands, underline the importance of financial obstacles to accessing employment, particularly fear of losing disabilities pensions and not maintaining current living conditions. The notion of social inclusion puts into question longstanding institutions such as rehabilitative day centres or sheltered workshops (Albin et al. 1994, Block 1993). In studies comparing new SE models with sheltered work methods, traditional rehabilitation or day care, the SE methods produce positive employment outcomes without ill effects on clients' health (Becker et al. 2001, Drake et al. 1996b, Oldman et al. 2005). In spite of these findings, mental health professionals are still often seen as discouraging people from seeking competitive employment, for fear of negative consequences on clients' health (Office of the Deputy Prime Minister 2004).

In short, institutional solutions creating protective comfort zones such as extensive disabilities benefits, day centres and sheltered workshops can paradoxically – by the dependence they induce – become obstacles to accessing and maintaining competitive employment in the community. Yesterday's solutions become today's problems.

Obstacles and facilitators at the macrosocial level

Although employers can be welcoming to people with disabilities (Hagner and Cooney 2003), discrimination encountered within the labour market is real (Scheid 2005). Small business owners questioned about hiring people with mental illness worry about their social and emotional skills (Hand and Tryssenaar 2006). Weighing the benefits and risks of disclosure of psychiatric disabilities to an employer is a difficult task (MacDonald-Wilson 2005). Furthermore, internalised stigma is a significant issue in people with mental health difficulties, many of whom believe they have no chance of obtaining employment (Thornicroft 2006). And few do. A 12-country European comparison showed that although employment rates of people with schizophrenia are related to macroeconomic indicators such as the general employment rate, taxes and social benefits, there seems to be little link to gross domestic product or active labour market policy (Kilian and Becker 2007). Even though higher local unemployment rates do predict SE programme outcomes (Becker et al. 2006), with for example rural centres in certain studies attaining high employment rates than urban centres (Drake et al. 1998), this influence is not prohibitive (Bond et al. 2008). IPS programmes in Europe have been found to produce systematically positive results in countries with varying unemployment rates (Burns et al. 2007, 2008).

In summary, discrimination against people with mental health problems and consequent internalised stigmatisation are in all likelihood more important obstacles to accessing learning and employment than macroeconomic factors such as gross domestic product or population unemployment rates.

Method

In the EMILIA Project, data were collected at eight demonstration sites (see Table 8.1) in Paris, France; Tuzla, Bosnia-Herzegovina; Zealand, Denmark; London, UK; Athens, Greece; Warsaw, Poland; Barcelona, Spain; and Bodø, Norway.

Table 8.1 Organisations participating in the EMILIA Project at the eight European sites

Athens, Greece: EPAPSY, an NGO running a Day Centre in Athens and a Mobile Mental Health Unit in the Cycladic Islands and a network of local authorities and other mental health agencies involved in creating a social cooperative.

Barcelona, Spain: The Mental Health Outpatient Unit and the Forum Day Hospital in the Hospital del Mar working in conjunction with JOIA, a Recovery and Social Integration NGO, and ADDEM, a mental health service-user organisation

Bodø, Norway: Rehabilitation and assertive outreach teams of the Nordland Psychiatric Hospital;

London, UK: the Mental Health and Social Work Department of the School for Health and Social Sciences of Middlesex University in London, working in conjunction with user organisations and user consultants.

Paris, France: Secteur Flandre, a Community Mental Health Centre in central Paris, working in conjunction with the Maison Blanche Research Laboratory, two user NGOs, an information and resource centre about work, training and jobs (la Cité des Métiers) and professional and vocational integration structures.

Zealand, Denmark: The Department of Education, Development and Research in the Storstrom County Psychiatric Services in conjunction with rehabilitation centres with a specific peer-support worker approach

Tuzla, Bosnia: The Psychiatric Clinic in the city of Tuzla, working in conjunction with the user organisation 'Feniks' and the Research Department of HealthNet International (HNI), an NGO providing consultancy services for mental health care.

Warsaw, Poland: A community team and day centre within the Psychiatry and Neurology Institute working together with a clubhouse NGO in Warsaw (Fountain House).

In each site, the attempt was made to provide access to lifelong learning and employment or significant activities in the mental health area to people with serious and enduring mental illness. The resulting eight case studies included an obstacles and facilitators monitoring process, designed to optimise inter-site programme fidelity and share solutions found for overcoming obstacles on both organisational and individual levels using a specific survey feedback instrument, the *EMILIA Guidebook to Supporting Users in Learning and Vocational Integration*, posted on the project's internal website in September 2006. The Guidebook, constantly updated throughout the 54 month project, was a living document designed to help demonstration sites learn from each other's experience, from other partners and from the scientific literature about the obstacles organisations and users encounter and the solutions they find to these problems throughout the project. The monitoring process involved all sites responding to seven consecutive surveys with three project stakeholder groups (researchers, health and social care professionals, users) with results published on the EMILIA website and accessible to all partners. The current paper describes the principle individual and institutional obstacles encountered at the eight European sites and the solutions found.

Three surveys took place before users began training and accessing employment, three during project implementation with users and one as users completed final interviews at the end of project implementation (Table 8.2).

The monitoring process described in the current paper used a qualitative, research-action approach, with researchers from each site regularly feeding information on obstacles encountered into a jointly run Obstacles and Solutions Monitoring tool on the Internet.

Results

The monitoring process drew on survey information from each of the eight sites at seven different points during the research-action, grouping obstacles into three broad categories: individual, institutional and macrosocial. The results presented in the current paper describe the different obstacles observed at the eight sites for each of these categories.

Individual level obstacles and solutions

Throughout the EMILIA monitoring process, problems at the individual level were a recurrent but low profile theme. Trainers and certain users regularly mentioned cognitive difficulties maintaining concentration or keeping up with other participants during collective training sessions. Symptom management could be an issue both for the individual with the symptom, the trainer or vocational worker, and the other members of the group in training sessions. For many, mental illness was not their only problem. Physical health problems, substance misuse, problems in their personal lives, and social and housing problems had a major impact on learning and employment participation and plans.

Gaining self-esteem, having confidence in their personal skills and their ability to succeed were frequently mentioned, particularly by the users themselves. Fear of failure can be debilitating. Trainers underlined the importance of allowing participants to test out new ideas, to make mistakes, to say 'I don't know', to joke. Building on existing skills, but

Table 8.2 Seven consecutive surveys on obstacles and facilitators encountered before and during implementation

Prior to implementation	
1: May 2006	Email questionnaire to site leaders on the history of training and employing users at each site, current practices, experience with peer support, current access to information and lifelong learning for users and potential obstacles to implementation.
2: Sept 2006	Face-to-face interviews with site leaders on obstacles actually encountered in setting up the project at their site.
3: Nov 2006	Email questionnaire to site leaders asking them to obtain information from local social work and job integration professionals concerning the existence, at their site, of obstacles identified in the scientific literature.
During implementation	
4: Nov 2007	Face-to-face interviews with site researchers on obstacles that institutions and the first three users had encountered during the initial implementation phase and the solutions found.
5: Jan–March 2008	Site researchers completed one questionnaire for each training package used during the first phase of implementation, describing the obstacles encountered during training and the solutions found.
6: June 2008	Email questionnaire to site researchers followed up by back-up telephone interviews on user access to employment or significant activities during the first year of EMILIA implementation.
At the close of the project	
7: May 2009	Email questionnaire to site researchers and three users at each site on obstacles encountered and solutions found in maintaining integrated educational and SE systems at each site.

also acquiring new knowledge and skills, were key to success. Indeed, many users lacked experience with organised training, with several reporting that participating in EMILIA training was not easy, especially at the beginning. Receiving support from trainers was essential. Other perceived the lack of work experience as a major handicap. Professionals underlined issues related to user motivation, particularly during periods of inactivity. Insufficient social skills and difficulty functioning in large groups came up frequently in the monitoring process, and were often associated with a lack of social support. Being able to count on a social network can be essential not only for psychological reasons but also quite simply to find work.

The themes of recovery and empowerment, often relatively new to European mental health services, became increasingly present as the project moved forward, the recovery training module being particularly successful across all sites. In the EMILIA training modules, being part of a group of people with common aims gave users the opportunity to reflect on common issues. Sharing opinions with other people who want to access learning or work is a major step in gaining a perspective on one's own situation, particularly with regard to questions of symptom management and internalised stigma.

Asked to describe the principle strengths of the first three users at each of the eight sites, researchers distinguished between personal strengths such as knowing your strengths and weaknesses (8), being self-confident (6), being in good health (3), being motivated (3) and having skills (2) – and social strengths such as being able to rely on the local Emilia team (8), having a social or support network that you can count on (5) and wanting to play an active role in society (4).

The main solutions at the individual level would seem to be to encourage strengths-building approaches within a recovery framework and with appropriate support: understanding one's own strengths and being able to rely on both the group and the EMILIA professionals for support were key to success.

Institutional level obstacles and solutions

Disability benefits and other social allocations

The criteria for inclusion in the EMILIA project were mental health service users with a history of long-term mental illness, aged 18–64, with a diagnosis of schizophrenia F20 (ICD-10), schizoaffective disorder F25 (ICD-10) or bipolar disorder F30-F31 (ICD-10) and at least three years of using mental health services. It is thus not surprising that almost all participants at the beginning of the study were receiving disabilities benefits of various sorts. The risk or fear of the user losing their disability benefits when accessing lifelong learning and employment was identified by the users themselves as a significant obstacle. This risk or perception of risk was also an issue for families, some of whom depended on the user's benefits from a financial point of view.

Social work professionals at all sites underlined the fact that applying for benefits takes considerable time and effort. According to these professionals, most ground-level stakeholders (users, informal carers, families, healthcare professionals, key workers and social workers) end up being reluctant to take the risk of upsetting the boat – whether they fully understand the rules or not. Fear of having to go through this process again is a major obstacle for both the user and for their family, and this fear is often present regardless of the reality of the risk or the existence of any compensatory systems put into place to obviate income loss. In almost all participating countries, it is possible to suspend benefits temporarily in one way or another, thus allowing the person to experiment getting a job. However, across Europe, the social welfare systems are often so complex that users need to have access to social work expertise – or develop that expertise themselves – in order to profit from the system. For example, in certain cases in France, administrative solutions to facilitate the vocational inclusion process by removing the risk of losing disabilities benefits are held in check by the risks linked to other social welfare benefits. Getting a paid job reduces the right to many allocations and therefore creates a real and significant risk of economic difficulties should the employment attempt not be successful.

Such institutional obstacles often have extended microsocial ramifications. The consequences for the families and carers of people with disabilities must also be taken into account. The various benefits and allocations of a family member with mental illness can be a major source of income for the entire family. If the person tries to work and loses these pensions, this constitutes a risk for the entire family.

Corrective mechanisms aimed at countering perverse effects of disabilities benefits

Although compensatory and incentive systems for training and employing people with disabilities exist across Europe, for a multitude of reasons, in many situations, they have little effect on the social inclusion of people with severe and enduring mental illness. To combat the tendency for institutional support for people with disabilities to paradoxically encourage social isolation or exclusion, many countries have put into place corrective institutional mechanisms. For example, in no country is a disabilities pension an obstacle to accessing training (with the partial exception of Spain, where service users who have a total disability allowance would have to pay if they wanted to access any form of training). On a more proactive level, all countries, with the exception of Greece and Norway, have created a special 'disabled worker' status that gives people with disabilities who work special advantages that might make it more attractive for them to work or to remain working. Furthermore, incentives for employers to employ people with disabilities – or fines if they do not – are frequent across Europe. Typically, this involves a certain proportion of the workforce or the workforce budget being used to employ people with disabilities. Unfortunately, in most countries, although these laws exist, they often have little real impact on actually integrating people with mental health disabilities into the competitive workforce. In certain countries, employers can fulfil their obligations by, for example, outsourcing to sheltered workshops. In many cases, social workers report employers favouring other categories of disabled people, considered more 'functional' and perceived of as being easier to integrate than people with severe psychological problems.

Sheltered work

In most countries, the traditional solution to the vocational aspirations of people with mental health disabilities has been the sheltered workshop system, which provides work for people with disabilities outside of the competitive job market – although, in the former communist countries, these are 'dying out' (Warsaw) or 'largely extinct' (Tuzla) in so far as people with serious and enduring mental illness are concerned. Although these sheltered work systems were put into place as a first stepping-stone towards integration into real-world employment, social workers at EMILIA sites report that, once users are admitted to the system, they tend to stay there until they retire.

Lack of experience and expertise in providing lifelong learning for users

Training users in groups is rare in mental healthcare delivery – and this was certainly true at the eight EMILIA demonstration sites. Before implementation, although all sites that were mental health service providers were providing training on developing specific, practical, everyday living skills such as knitting, swimming, football, cooking, shopping or cleaning, this is mostly done on an individual case management level within a rehabilitation service framework. Furthermore, group training in psycho-education is not the general rule, information on mental illness being given in one-to-one sessions as part of general healthcare delivery. Only four of the eight demonstration sites were proposing any form of group training and, of these, only Barcelona and Warsaw were providing training for users or for professionals with the aim of helping users to develop skills for the competitive working world. The whole idea of offering users training in group sessions without a specifically therapeutic objective constituted for many sites a cultural revolution, requiring careful monitoring.

Little experience and administrative difficulties employing users

Site researchers' reviews of the history of user employment in each institution showed that user employment by psychiatric hospitals was common until fairly late in the twentieth century. Then, specific regulations just prior to the deinstitutionalisation period were introduced to reinforce the notion that psychiatric hospitals are to provide care and not long-term social services. Making patients work became stigmatised as exploitation of people with serious mental illness. A prevailing theme throughout the monitoring process was staff reticence to encourage users to work for fear of relapse, a theme often linked to staff resistance to users playing a role in the health care system in general. Local steering groups therefore underlined the importance of involving all stakeholders as early as possible in the planning process.

Actually employing people without accredited diplomas is problematic in many countries. Obtaining accreditation for EMILIA training modules was a significant challenge. Although the specific training modules developed by the project brought trainees new skills, only Middlesex University was able to provide some form of formal accreditation.

Three demonstration sites (Athens, Paris and Warsaw) and two non-demonstration site partners (Ljubljana and Vilnius) had set up or helped set up profit-making or non-profit-making enterprises, where their institution is not the employer, with the specific aim of employing either their own users or other people with serious ongoing mental illness. None of these organisations provided work in the area of mental health. Four sites had services whose specific aim was to help people with mental health problems to keep their job (other than therapeutic sessions that may help indirectly):

- creating support networks between the health provider and the workplace (sheltered workshops) (Barcelona)
- training with the aim of keeping a job (Warsaw)
- concurrent training and placement (Aarhus)
- mentors (Ljubljana).

Lack of personnel and resources

At several sites, although their mission includes helping users access supported employment, existing social work staff spent all of their time on activities such as finding housing, organising disabilities allowances, paying bills or obtaining residential permits. Helping users find jobs, although considered important, is simply lower down on the list of essential priorities. Having human resources with a specific social inclusion, supported education and employment remit are a priority.

Macrosocial level obstacles and solutions

Increasingly competitive job markets in contexts of high general population unemployment as well as the accumulation for many users of several sources of potential discrimination (such as mental illness, gender, age or ethnicity) create significant barriers that, in most European countries, have necessitated putting into place major policy mechanisms to compensate employers, combat discrimination and provide incentive systems for workforce inclusion initiatives. The specific problems of former communist countries with a rapid transition from theoretically full employment – including employment of people with disabilities – to the competitive job market, must be underlined. In many cases, historical institutional solutions to problems relating to mental illness and disabilities have often in turn become obstacles to social inclusion in general and integrating education and competitive employment in particular. Dismantling these institutional obstacles and fighting against stigma and discrimination when reintegrating people into the community can be a daunting process both on individual and institutional levels.

Stigma and discrimination against people with mental health problems

Demonstration sites emphasised the effects of discrimination, stigma and internalised stigma on both users and their families. In the final survey, when asked what advice they would give to the authorities in their country to help people with mental illness access training and jobs, the users themselves underlined the importance of fighting against discrimination and stigma. Resistance to social inclusion does not come from employers alone. At one site, a local job centre refused to publish an advertisement seeking people with a user background on the grounds that such people were ill, could not work and therefore that it was not ethically correct. Researchers at two sites mentioned social work professionals being overly protective or pessimistic, considering the competitive job market – and in some cases even the sheltered workshop job market – as being too harsh, too heartless or too stigmatising for their clients. In sites like Paris, for example, the disability status itself is perceived by both users and professionals as creating a risk for discrimination.

Considerable site differences appear with regard to users' family situations. Although at most EMILIA sites, many users were living independently, in countries such as Greece, Spain and Poland, the vast majority of users were living with their family of origin. Many of these families had been keeping their mentally ill family member at home for many years. Due to social stigma, certain families can be reticent to allow the mentally ill person to leave home, to look for a job and risk bringing shame onto the family. Families often have trouble believing that the mentally ill are able to work or that this should be a desirable aim.

High local unemployment rates

In Warsaw and Tuzla, with unemployment rates of 15% and 45% respectively, researchers considered that people with mental health problems would not stand a chance on the competitive job market. As the project moved forward, the 2008–9 economic crisis added to this already difficult situation.

Illegal or undeclared work

In the initial survey, existing black market or undeclared work was considered a potential obstacle for implementing the project, should candidates be unwilling to declare this and therefore risk losing income, albeit illegal, when integrating the EMILIA process. However, during the project, although some sites give examples of people with mental health disabilities working illegally or working informally, typically within their family, this proved to be rare and of an irregular nature.

The PRET and SIRC implementation checklists

In the monitoring process described in the current paper, researchers from each site regularly fed information on obstacles encountered and solutions found into a jointly run Obstacles and Solutions Monitoring Checklist on the project website. For each obstacle encountered at any research site, solutions used or envisaged were shared with all partners, whether they were on an institutional project implementation level or concerning an individual action plan. Ten months into the project, the monitoring checklist was converted into two separate implementation instruments: the Pathways Readiness Evaluation Tool (PRET) and the Services and Institutions Readiness Checklist (SIRC).

The PRET is a simple three column checklist to be used by each user both before and during EMILIA-type projects to help them build individual lifelong learning and employment plans. For each plan, users and their support workers check the issues in the left-hand column to see whether they personally might be concerned. The middle column lists solutions used or envisaged by users or care providers that have already confronted these issues. The right hand column gives references to training programmes, professional skills or publications that might be of help. The PRET tool is divided into five main sections: Illness and Disability Issues, Individual Knowledge, Skills and Means, Inertia related to current personal social situation, Microsocial Issues (family, network and support) and Employer/Employment Issues. Table 8.3 gives examples of PRET checklist items drawn from different sections.

The second tool, the Services and Institutions Readiness Checklist (SIRC), initially based on obstacles and solutions described in the scientific literature, was designed be used by the demonstration sites in the EMILIA project as sites began implementation. The SIRC was considerably extended throughout implementation to include obstacles and facilitators encountered by individual sites throughout the EMILIA project, allowing thus a sharing of experience between sites and a corresponding optimisation of the EMILIA process. When envisaging an EMILIA-type user empowerment project, organisations are invited to check the issues in the left-hand column to see whether their

Table 8.3   Examples of Pathways Readiness Evaluation Tool (PRET) checklist items

Issue	Solution used or envisaged	Contact/reference
The 'official' mental illness is not the only mental health problem. Co-existing drug & alcohol problems.	Build personal development plan around all personal issues.	Use EMILIA training module: *Drugs and Alcohol*/Contingency Management: reinforce desired behaviours, control attendance, reduce substance abuse (Drebing 2006)
Family depends on grants	Working with the families from the start	Integrate local carer organisations into steering group
	Find solution to family problems	Consult social worker
Family unable to imagine the user working; negative beliefs & attitudes	Working with the families to encourage positive beliefs & attitudes	Use EMILIA training module: Supporting Someone Close

Note: The complete PRET checklist can be accessed at www.entermentalhealth.com.

Table 8.4 Examples from the Services and Institutions Readiness Checklist (SIRC)

Issue	Solution used or envisaged	Contact/reference
Statutory legitimacy to train users: some healthcare institutions have no mandate to train users (so they cannot use their funds to do this)	Produce evidence that social inclusion will significantly reduce use of services. Engage authorities in a research and development strategy to investigate this. Convince authorities to support lifelong learning activities for mental health users by funding an NGO to do the training.	Contact outside NGOs or other organisations to provide LLL within the health system if impossible in health system. See ENTER Mental Health Website for access to free online training modules in many European languages.
Impossible to employ people who do not possess specific diplomas within statutory mental health services	Investigate possibility of creating links with a teaching institution to get accreditation for EMILIA-type modules. Study legal texts governing accreditation in your country.	Consult social workers, jurists
Staff having difficulty imagining the person working	Integrate users and independent ethics consultants into recruitment panel	Make sure professionals with user experience are members of the Steering Committee, with the staff in question

Note: The complete SIRC checklist can be accessed at www.entermentalhealth.com.

institution could be concerned. The middle column describes solutions used or envisaged by sites in the EMILIA Project that have already confronted these issues or by similar lifelong learning/employment projects described in the literature. The right hand column gives references to training programmes, professional skills or bibliographical references. The SIRC instrument is in three sections: (1) institutional issues, (2) macrosocial issues, (3) project methodology issues. Table 8.4 gives examples of SIRC checklist items drawn from the three different sections.

Conclusions

The obstacles monitoring process used in the 54 month EMILIA project has shown how barriers for people with serious mental illness to accessing training, employment and social inclusion can be encountered and resolved from individual through to institutional and macrosocial levels. However findings also underline the importance of identifying not only obstacles and facilitators for the individual but also for the organisation that wishes to set up projects aiming at user empowerment and social inclusion through lifelong learning and employment. The resulting PRET and SIRC instruments are potentially valuable outcomes for future efforts to design both individual and institutional projects in this area.

References

Albin, J. M., Rhodes, L. and Mank, D. (1994). 'Realigning Organizational Culture, Resources, and Community Roles: Changeover to Community Employment', *Journal of the Association for Persons with Severe Handicaps*, IX(2), 105–15.

Australian Bureau of Statistics (2008). *National Survey of Mental Health and Wellbeing: Summary of Results, 2007* (Canberra, Commonwealth of Australia).

Baron, R. and Salzer, M. S. (2000). 'The Career Patterns of Persons with Serious Mental Illness: Generating a New Vision of Lifetime Careers for Those in Recovery', *Psychiatric Rehabilitation Skills* IV, 136–56.

Becker, D. R., Xie, H., McHugo, G. J., Halliday, J. and Martinez, R. A. (2006). 'What Predicts Supported Employment Program Outcomes?', *Community Mental Health Journal* XLII(3), 303–13.

Becker, D. R., Smith, J., Tanzman, B., Drake, R. E. and Tremblay, T. (2001). 'Fidelity of Supported Employment Programs and Employment Outcomes', *Psychiatric Services*, XXVIII, 834–6.

Becker, D., Whitley, R., Bailey, E. L. and Drake, R. E. (2007). 'Long-Term Employment Trajectories among Participants with Severe Mental Illness in Supported Employment', *Psychiatric Services*, LVIII(7), 922–8.

Berthoud, R. (2006). *The Employment Rates of Disabled People* (London: Department of Work and Pensions).

Block, L. (1993). 'Saying Goodbye to an Old Friend: The Closure of a Sheltered Workshop', *Canadian Journal of Rehabilitation*, VII(2), 111–18.

Bond, G. R., Drake, R. E. and Becker, D. R. (2008). 'An Update on Randomized Controlled Trials of Evidence-Based Supported Employment', *Psychiatric Rehabilitation Journal*, XXXI, 280–9.

Bond, G. R., Becker, D. R., Drake, R. E., Rapp, C., Meisler, N., Lehman, A. F., Bell, M. D. and Blyler, C. R. (2001). 'Implementing Supported Employment as an Evidence-Based Practice', *Psychiatric Services*, LII, 313–22. http://psychservices. psychiatryonline.org/cgi/reprint/52/3/313, date accessed 14 June 2011.

Bond, G. R., Xie, H. and Drake, R. E. (2007). 'Can SSDI and SSI Beneficiaries with Mental Illness Benefit From Evidence-Based Supported Employment?' *Psychiatric Services*, LVIII(11), 1412–20.

Burns, T., Catty, J., Becker, T., Drake, R. E., Fioritti, A., Knapp, M., Lauber, C., Rössler, W., Tomov, T., van Busschbach, J., White, S. D., Wiersma, D. and EQOLISE Group (2007). 'The Effectiveness of Supported Employment for People with Severe Mental Illness: A Randomised Controlled Trial', *Lancet*, CCCLXX(9593), 1146–52.

Burns, T., White, S. J., Catty, J. and EQOLISE group (2008). 'Individual Placement and Support in Europe: the EQOLISE trial. International', *Review of Psychiatry*, XX(6), 498–502.

Burns, T., Catty, J., White, S., Becker, T., Koletsi, M., Fioritti, A., Rossler, W., Tomov, T., van Busschbach, J., Wiersma, D., Lauber, C. and EQOLISE group (2009). 'The Impact of Supported Employment and Working on Clinical and Social Functioning: Results of an International Study of Individual Placement and Support', *Schizophrenia Bulletin*, XXXV(5), 949–58.

Campbell, K., Bond, G. R., Drake, R. E., McHugo, G. J. and Xie, H. (2010) Client predictors of employment outcomes in high-fidelity supported employment: a regression analysis. *The Journal of Nervous and Mental Disease* 198(8), 556–63.

Catty, J., Lissouba, P., White, S., Becker, T., Drake, R. E., Fioritti, A., Knapp, M., Lauber, C., Rossler, W., Tomov, T., van Busschbach, J., Wiersma, D., Burns, T. and EQOLISE group (2008). 'Predictors of Employment for People with Severe Mental Illness: Results of an International Six-Centre Randomised Controlled Trial', *The British Journal of Psychiatry*, CXCII(3), 224–31.

Collins, M. E., Mowbray, C. T. and Bybee, D. (2000). 'Characteristics Predicting Successful Outcomes of Participants with Severe Mental Illness in Supported Education', *Psychiatric Services*, LI, 774–80.

Collins, M. E., Bybee, D. and Mowbray, C. T. (1998). 'Effectiveness of Supported Education for Individuals with Psychiatric Disabilities: Results from and Experimental Study', *Community Mental Health Journal*, XXXIV, 595–613.

Council of the European Union (2000), *Presidency Conclusions, 23 and 24 March*. Lisbon: European Council. http://www.consilium.europa.eu/uedocs/cms_data/docs/pressdata/en/ec/00100-r1.en0.htm, date accessed 15 December 2011.

Danley, K. (1997). 'Long-Term Outcomes of Participants in a Career Education Program for Young Adults Who Have Psychiatric Disabilities' *Briefing paper No. 1 of 3* (Boston, Mass: Boston University Center for Psychiatric Rehabilitation).

Drake, R. E., McHugo, G. J., Becker, D. R., Anthony, W. A. and Clark, R. E. (1996a) 'The New Hampshire Study of Supported Employment for People with Severe Mental Illness: Vocational Outcomes', *Journal of Consulting and Clinical Psychology*, LXIV, 391–9.

Drake, R. E., Becker, D. R., Biesanz, J. C., Wyzik, P. F. and Torrey, W. C. (1996b). 'Day Treatment versus Supported Employment for Persons with Severe Mental Illness: A Replication Study', *Psychiatric Services*, XLVII(10), 1125–7.

Drake, R. E., Fox, T. S., Leather, P. K., Becker, D. R., Musumeci, J. S., Ingram, W. F. and McHugo, G. J. (1998). 'Regional Variation in Competitive Employment for Persons with Severe Mental Illness', *Administration and Policy in Mental Health and Mental Health Services Research*, XXV(5): 493–504.

Drake, R. E. and Bond, G. R. (2008). 'The Future of Supported Employment for People with Severe Mental Illness', *Psychiatric Rehabilitation Journal*, XXXI: 367–76.

Gilson, S. F. (1998). 'Case Management and Supported Employment: A Good Fit', *Journal of Case Management*, VII(1), 10–17.

Gioia, D. (2005). 'Career Development in Schizophrenia: A Heuristic Framework', *Community Mental Health Journal*, XLI(3), 307–25.

Hagner, D. and Cooney, B. (2003). 'Building Employer Capacity to Support Employees with Severe Disabilities in the Workplace', *Work* XXI(1), 77–82.

Hand, C. and Tryssenaar, J. (2006). 'Small Business Employers' Views on Hiring Individuals with Mental Illness', *Psychiatric Rehabilitation Journal*, XXIX(3), 166–73.

Howard, L. M., Heslin, M., Leese, M., McCrone, P., Rice, C., Jarrett, M. and Spokes, T. (2010). 'Supported Employment: Randomised Controlled Trial', *The British Journal of Psychiatry* CXCVI, 404–11.

Isenwater, W., Lanham, W. and Thornhill, H. (2002). 'The College Link Program: Evaluation of a Supported Education Initiative in Great Britain', *Psychosocial Rehabilitation Journal*, XXVI(1), 43–50.

Kanter, J. (2008). 'Employment Outcomes for SSA Beneficiaries', *Psychiatric Services*, LIX, 114–5. http://psychservices.psychiatryonline.org/cgi/content/full/59/1/114, date accessed 14 June 2011.

Kilian, R. and Becker, T. (2007). 'Macro-Economic Indicators and Labour Force Participation of People with Schizophrenia', *Journal of Mental Health*, XVI(2), 211–22.

Kirsner, J. (2009). 'Supported Education Services for Young People with Severe Mental Illness', Preliminary Report, Australasian Society for Psychiatric Research working party http://www.aspr.org.au/pdfs/Return%20to%20educati on%20for%20young%20people%20with%20severe%20mental%20illness.doc, date accessed 21 December 2011.

Liberman, R. P. (2008). 'Employment Outcomes for SSA Beneficiaries', *Psychiatric Services* LIX, 114–5.

Linhorst, D. M. (2006). *Empowering People with Severe Mental Illness: A Practical Guide* (Oxford: Oxford University Press).

MacDonald-Wilson, K. L. (2005). 'Managing Disclosure of Psychiatric Disabilities to Employers', *Journal of Applied Rehabilitation Counseling. Special Issue: Psychiatric Rehabilitation*, XXXVI(4), 11–21.

Marwaha, S. and Johnson, S. (2004). 'Schizophrenia and Employment: A Review', *Social Psychiatry and Psychiatric Epidemiology*, XXXIX, 337–49.

McGurk, S. R., Mueser, K T., Harvey, P. D., LaPuglia, R. and Marder, J. (2003) 'Cognitive and Symptom Predictors of Work Outcomes for Clients with Schizophrenia in Supported Employment', *Psychiatric Services*, LIV(8), 1129–35.

McGurk, S. R., Mueser, K. T., Feldman, K., Wolfe, A. R. and Pascaris, A. (2007). 'Cognitive Training for Supported Employment: 2–3 Year Outcomes of a Randomized Controlled Trial', *American Journal of Psychiatry*, CLXIV(3), 437–41.

Mowbray, C., Collins, M. and Bybee, D. (1999). 'Supported Education for Individuals with Psychiatric Disabilities: Long-Term Outcomes from an Experimental Study', *Social Work Research*, XXIII(2), 89–100.

Mowbray, C. T., Collins, M. E., Bellamy, C. D., Megivern, D. A., Bybee, D. and Szilvagyi, S. (2005). 'Supported Education for Adults with Psychiatric Disabilities: An Innovation for Social Work and Psychosocial Rehabilitation Practice', *Social Work*, L(1), 7–20. PMID: 15688676.

Mueser, K. T., Becker, D. R. and Wolfe, R. (2001). 'Supported Employment, Job Preferences, Job Tenure and Satisfaction', *Journal of Mental Health*, X, 411–17.

Office of the Deputy Prime Minister (2004). *Mental Health and Social Exclusion* (Social Exclusion Unit Report, London).

Ogunleye, J. (2009). 'Lifelong Learning Provision for Mental Health Service Users: An EMILIA Research Report on Disparities, Similarities and a Common European Social Policy Agenda' in N. Popov, C. Wolhuter, B. Leutwyler and J. Ogunleye (eds). *Teacher Training, Education Policy and Social Inclusion*, VII (Sofia, Bulgaria: Bureau for Educational Services), 281–5.

Oldman, J., Thomson, L., Calsaferri, K., Luke, A. and Bond, G. R. (2005). 'A Case Report of the Conversion of Sheltered Employment to Evidence-Based Supported Employment in Canada', *Psychiatric Services*, LVI(11), 1436–40.

Pallisera, M., Vila, M. and Valls, M. J. (2003). 'The Current Situation of Supported Employment in Spain: Analysis and Perspectives Based on the Perception of Professionals', *Disability and Society*, XVIII(6), 797–810.

Razzano, L. A., Cook, J. A., Burke-Miller, J. K., Mueser, K. T., Pickett-Schenk, S. A., Grey, D. D., Goldberg, R. W., Blyler, C. R., Gold, P. B., Leff, H. S., Lehman, A. F., Shafer, M. S., Blankertz, L. E., McFarlane, W. R., Toprac, M. G., Ann Carey, M. (2005). 'Clinical Factors Associated with Employment among People with Severe Mental Illness: Findings from the Employment Intervention Demonstration Program', *Journal of Nervous and Mental Disease*, CXCIII(11), 705–13.

Scheid, T. L. (2005). 'Stigma as a Barrier to Employment: Mental Disability and the Americans with Disabilities Act', *International Journal of Law and Psychiatry*, XVIII(6), 670–90.

Schneider, J., Slade, J., Secker, J., Rinaldi, M., Boyce, M., Johnson, R., Floyd, M. and Grove, B. (2009). 'SESAMI Study of Employment Support for People with Severe Mental Health Problems: 12-Month Outcomes', XVII(2), 151–8.

Smith, A. and Twomey, B. (2002). 'Labour Market Experiences of People with Disabilities', *Labour Market Trends*, August: 415–27.

Thornicroft, G. (2006). *Actions Speak Louder: Tackling Discrimination against People with Mental Illness* (London: Mental Health Foundation).

Tsang, H. W. H. (2008). 'Enhancing Employment Opportunities of People with Mental Illness through an Integrated Supported Employment approach of Individual Placement and Support and Social Skills Training', *Hong Kong Medical Journal*, XIV(3), 41–6.

Van Erp, N. H. J., Giesen, F. B. M., van Weeghel, J. et al. (2007). 'A Multi-Site Study of Implementing Supported Employment in the Netherlands' *Psychiatric Services*, LVIII, 1421–6.

Waghorn, G., Chant, D. and Whiteford, H. (2003). 'The Strength of Self-Reported Course of Illness in Predicting Vocational Recovery for Persons with Schizophrenia', *Journal of Vocational Rehabilitation*, XVIII, 33–41.

Wehmanand, P. and Revell, G. (2005). 'Lessons Learned from the Provision and Funding of Employment Services for the MR/DD Population: Implications for Assessing the Adequacy of the SSA Ticket to Work', *Journal of Disability Policy Studies*, vol. 16, no. 2, 84–101.

Part III

Empowerment and Lifelong Learning

9
Empowerment: Key Concepts and Evidence Base

Peter Ryan, Anja Esther Baumann and Chris Griffiths

Introduction

This chapter seeks to clarify the nature of the term empowerment, to review the policy context and evidence base concerning the impact of empowerment upon mental health service users, and to explore implications at mental health service level. Historically, people with mental health problems did not have a voice either in society as a whole or within mental health services; they and their families were not involved in decision-making processes in policy and practice of mental health services, and they had to face social exclusion and discrimination in many facets of life. Current reports on mental health in the European region show that this has not changed significantly in recent years (WHO 2009). Disempowerment of mental health services users has operated at a variety of levels, ranging from the societal/structural to the individual levels. At the individual level, through a process of internalisation of the external stigma, many service users remain traumatised for long periods of time with damaged internal senses of identity, self-efficacy and self-worth through their difficult experience of living in society with a mental illness. Self-stigma of mental health service users has been shown to be inversely proportion to empowerment (Brohan et al. 2011). With respect to their experiences of mental health services, it is often the case that they are generally poorly informed, and often poorly consulted or poorly treated by mental health services. At the societal/structural level, stigma against mental illness is universally present in all societies, with numerous barriers to accessing work and other social activities.

Definition of empowerment

In terms of a basic definition of the term 'empowerment', there is a considerable diversity of approach. The United Nations places emphasis on participation in its definition of empowerment, stating that:

> Development must be by the people, not only for them. People must participate fully in the decisions and processes that shape their lives.
>
> (UNDP 1995, p. 12)

The EU underlines the notion of people having the means to take responsible decisions:

> The process of granting people the power to take responsible initiatives to shape their own life and that of their community or society in economic, social and political terms.
>
> (EU COM 2001)

Rowlands (1995) emphasises that empowerment is multi-dimensional, and is therefore about much more than including access to decision–making with respect to mental health services for individuals. It also involves a 'paradigm shift' for mental health professionals, towards seeing service users as partners and collaborators. Blakemore (2003, p. 261) defines empowerment as:

> A process of change in which oppressed groups discover their ability to challenge those who oppress them. Empowerment can be brought about by change in the power structures which govern communities and social organisations.

Empowerment has therefore been used generically to describe situations of overcoming oppression or powerlessness experienced by stigmatised or marginalised groups – of which people with mental health difficulties are one.

Within the context of mental health services, there can be a misleading tendency to refer to empowerment purely in terms of issues of choice with respect to service use and contact with services. Whilst the degree of choice and control which the 'service user' can exercise with respect to the service is clearly crucial, issues of control and choice extend far more widely and embrace issues of power and control with respect to the broader society of which the 'service user' as citizen is a member, and how that citizenship can be exercised. In this broader societal context, empowerment refers to the level of choice, influence and control that mental health service users can exercise over all events in their lives. This is well summarised by Wallerstein (2006): 'The key to empowerment is the removal of formal or informal barriers and the transformation of power relations between individuals, communities, services and governments. Power is central to the idea of empowerment'.

Level of empowerment-and disempowerment

Historically, empowerment can be seen as occurring at three levels:

- Individual\psychological\interactional
- Influencing service provision and development
- Societal\structural.

It could be argued that a process of empowerment therefore needs to create an environment which takes onboard these three levels and needs to have in place specific steps and pathways that link these levels together.

Individual\psychological\interactional

At the individual level, empowerment is about increasing the capacity of individuals to become more self-reliant and is a means which allows increased participation in decisions, along with increased dignity and respect and a sense of belonging and contributing to a wider community.

Hope and respect

Hope is essential. A hopeful person believes in the possibility of future change and improvement; without hope, making an effort can seem pointless. Yet some professionals who label their patients incurable or chronic seem also to expect them to be motivated to take action and make changes in their lives, despite the overall hopelessness such labels convey. Showing respect to an individual is also vital. Carers need to show respect for the inherent dignity and individual autonomy of people with mental health problems, including acceptance of difference as part of human diversity and humanity (UN 2006).

Reclaiming one's life

As part of the process of psychiatric diagnosis and treatment, users and their families have often had their lives and their personal stories transformed into medical notes and case histories. Part of the empowerment process is therefore the reclaiming of these life stories. Similarly, the process of empowerment should include a reclaiming of one's sense of competence. In the early stages of participation in self-help groups, for example, members often tell one another their stories; both the act of telling and that of being listened to are important for group members. This can lead to a profound sense of self discovery that, despite traumatic and difficult experiences which may involve hospitalisation and all that this implies in terms of the dislocation of experience, it is possible to move onwards to an enhanced sense of self. This enhanced identity, encompassing the notion of recovery, does not deny the difficulties of having been mentally ill but, in an important sense, moves beyond them.

Feeling connected – not feeling alone

Empowerment does not happen to the individual alone, but has to do with experiencing a sense of shared experience through connectedness with other people. Often the most powerful social context for this can be in service-user groups operating outside of the context of mental health services. These service-user groups are often set up and run by service users themselves. The format of these organisations obviously depends on national and local culture and practice, varying for example from charities to social enterprises or co-operatives.

Growth and change that are never ending and self initiated

Empowerment is not a fixed destination, but a journey with many stages. No one reaches a final stage at which further empowerment is neither possible nor beneficial.

Decision-making power

Mental health professionals sometimes assume that service users and their families lack the ability to make decisions or to make 'correct' decisions. Services therefore sometimes adopt the paternalistic stance of limiting the number or quality of decisions that service users and families may make. Without support in making decisions, users are often maintained in long-term dependency relationships. People cannot become empowered and independent unless they are given the opportunity to make important decisions themselves about their lives.

In some circumstances, the barrier of denial of legal capacity is a key obstacle to decision-making: this legally prohibits people from making decisions. People with disabilities should enjoy legal capacity on an equal basis with others in all aspects of life, and states have an obligation to provide support to people who require assistance in making decisions (UN 2006).

Access to information and resources

Decision-making does not happen in a vacuum. The individual can make fair decisions only when he or she has sufficient information to weigh the possible consequences of various choices, to make informed decisions. Again, out of paternalism, mental health professionals sometimes restrict such information, believing restriction to be in the user's best interests. This can become a self-fulfilling prophecy: lacking adequate information, users may make choices that confirm professionals' beliefs in their inadequacy.

Having a range of options from which to choose

Meaningful choice means that users are offered and have the opportunity to explore the whole range of options that might be relevant, and receive any required and reasonable support to choose among them.

Learning skills that the individual defines as important

Health professionals sometimes complain that users have poor skills and seem unable to learn new one's. At the same time, the skills that professionals define as important are often not the one's that users find interesting or important. When users are given the opportunity to learn things that they want to learn they often surprise professionals (and sometimes themselves) by being able to learn them well. The EMILIA Project referred to in this book produces evidence that service users from very varied educational backgrounds do value lifelong learning, and are very keen to develop new skills which they themselves define as valuable for their own lives, particularly where these lead to greater social inclusion and employment opportunities of various kinds.

Societal\structural

At the societal\structural level, stigma is universally present in all societies and there are numerous barriers to full access to work and other normative social activities. Stigma is externally imposed through many different means and mechanisms in which the broader society expresses its prejudicial view that mental illness is in some deep sense problematic and needs somehow to be treated in isolation.

Understanding that people have rights

The self-help movement among mental health service users is part of a broader movement to establish basic human rights. There are parallels between this movement and other movements of oppressed and disadvantaged people, including racial and ethnic minorities, women, gay and lesbian people, and people with physical disabilities. The struggle for equal rights has been part of all these liberation movements. Through understanding their rights, people increase their sense of strength, self worth and self-confidence.

Moving from secrecy to transparency

People experiencing mental illness who can hide that fact often choose to do so, but this decision can take its toll in the form of decreased self-esteem and fear of discovery. Those who reach the point where they can reveal their identities as mental health service users are often more likely to display self-confidence. Services themselves need to be far more aware of the inherent stigmatising that can be part and parcel of receiving care. People can be helped to make decisions about disclosure through support in recognising that they have multiple characteristics, many of which are positive. It is also important for both people with mental health problems and society to recognise and accept that experience of mental health problems is a source of learning, growth and development, and it can bring additional knowledge, skills and qualities (WHO 2009).

The policy context and the research evidence base for empowerment

Policy context

Empowerment has been recognised as a core element of health promotion and disorder prevention in various international instruments such as the Ottawa Charter on Health Promotion (WHO 1986) and the Bangkok Charter for Health Promotion in a Globalized World (WHO 2005). In the 2005 Mental Health Action Plan for Europe, the World Health Organization European Member States agreed to ensure by 2010: 'representation of users and carers on committees and groups responsible for planning, delivering, reviewing and inspecting mental health activities' (WHO 2005). The implications of such user empowerment are not to be underestimated. Initial and essential steps in this direction have traditionally involved training professionals to help service users to access knowledge about their mental health problems, treatment and how to handle the mental and social healthcare systems. The WHO report on *Policies and practices for mental health in Europe – meeting the challenges* (WHO 2009) shows that users are represented on committees responsible for planning mental health services in less than half (48 per cent) of the 42 countries of the European Region which participated in the survey; even fewer countries (15 of 42) indicated that service users are represented on committees responsible for implementing policy on mental health services. Representation of service users and carers on inspection visits to mental health facilities, a commitment in the Mental Health Declaration for Europe (WHO 2005a), is far from standard in every part of the WHO European Region.

Evidence base for empowerment

There is some evidence that lack of influence or control can lead to poor health outcomes; conversely the ability to exercise control and influence, even where high stress is present, can act as a protective factor against levels of risk of cardio-vascular disease (Syme 1988; Tyers and Aston 2002). Also compatible with these findings is the literature on learned helplessness, which suggests that absence of influence or control can lead to the onset of depression (Garber and Seligman 1980). Disempowerment has therefore emerged as a key risk factor in the aetiology of disease. The corollary is that there is now a good deal of evidence from a number of different fields which suggest that empowerment is not 'just a set of values', but that in addition it leads to positive outcomes in care. These include: increased emotional well-being, independence, motivation to participate, and more effective coping strategies (Ryan and Deci 2000, Thompson and Soacapan 1991, Macleod and Nelson 2000).

Vauth et al. (2007) argue that the evaluative dimension of self-concept (self-efficacy and empowerment) mediates the psychological effects of self-stigmatising and coping with stigma. Measuring self-stigma and devaluation, coping with stigma, self-efficacy, empowerment, quality of life and depression in patients diagnosed with schizophrenia, their study found that over half of the empowerment reduction was explained by reduction in self-efficacy at dysfunctional coping level and higher levels of anticipated stigma. They concluded that an avoidant coping style is a risk factor for anticipatory stigma, which erodes self-efficacy and empowerment.

Some authors (Silver et al. 1986) have proposed that psychiatric symptoms can themselves be augmented by the negative and marginal social role occupied by severely mentally ill service users. Trainor and Trimblay (1992) found that active participation in self-help and mutual aid schemes was associated with lower rates of psychiatric admission and reduced usage of community mental health services. In a qualitative approach that generated service-user narratives, Nelson, Lord and Ochocka (2001) found that several strategies were cited by users as facilitating their recovery. These included

- Facilitated access to housing
- Financial assistance
- Choosing which services to receive
- Designing their own care plan
- A sense of meaningful involvement and participation in the services received.

Crane-Ross, Lutz and Roth (2006) defined service empowerment as 'the extent to which consumers participate in service decisions and the level of reciprocity and respect within the relationship with their case managers'. They examined the direct and indirect effects of service empowerment on four recovery outcomes: quality of life, level of functioning, self-reported symptomatology and service provider-reported symptomatology. They found that service-user perceptions of empowerment were the most powerful predictor of outcomes across the four outcomes. Jormfeldt et al. (2008) observed a direct link between levels of empowerment in people using mental health services and subjective ratings of health. Similarly, Barrett et al. (2010) found that mental health service-user empowerment mediated the relationship between treatment, and satisfaction with mental health services.

The strength of social networks has been found to be positively correlated with the empowerment of patients with schizophrenia living in the community (Bengtsson-Tops 2004). Using structural equation modelling to examine the impact of empowerment on the quality of life (QOL) of patients diagnosed with schizophrenia, Sibitz et al. (2011) found that the level of empowerment influenced QOL. The researchers reported that a poor social network contributed to a lack of empowerment and stigma, which resulted in depression and, in turn, in poor QOL. They concluded that mental health services focusing on the improvement of the social network, stigma reduction and especially on the development of empowerment, have the potential to reduce depression in patients with psychosis and improve their QOL.

Lecomte, Cy and Lesage (1999) observed an increase in active coping strategies for users in outpatient services who were involved in an empowerment based self-esteem group. A strengths approach can also enhance outcomes in the area of housing and independent living: Ware

(1999) found that service users in an innovative housing project which emphasised a strengths approach made significant progress towards independent living. The intervention emphasised group self-management, access to financial resources and reducing staffing levels.

Conclusion: making empowerment happen

Empowerment is complex and multi-dimensional. At the individual level, a process needs to be put into place in which individuals who have experienced mental illness can learn to develop their sense of self-determination, meaning and purpose, stemming from personal reflection upon understanding and acceptance of the events and experiences surrounding the events leading up to them becoming mentally ill, and their subsequent, potentially highly negative experience of services. Empowerment of a service user therefore involves a process of redefining and renegotiating self identity both with themselves, their relationship to mental health services and to society as a whole.

Mental health services have an important role to play in this process by restructuring themselves to address power imbalances between the service user, the practitioner, and the executive control of these services. At the societal and structural level, it also entails a more engaged stance with respect to wider society in terms of working actively with employers, for example to challenge stigma, and to assist in the renegotiation which the wider society needs to have with the mental health service user, as a citizen of society. A critical part of this broader social role is the value of human rights and dignity which is paramount in promoting equality and equity in rights and access to normally available social roles, opportunities and resources.

References

Bengtsson-Tops, A. (2004). 'Mastery in Patients with Schizophrenia Living in the Community: Relationship to Sociodemographic and Clinical Characteristics, Needs for Care and Support, and Social Network', *Journal of Psychiatric Mental Health Nursin*, XI, 298–304.

Barrett, B., Young, M. S., Teague, G. B., Winarski, J. T., Moore, K. A. and Ochshorn, E. (2010). 'Recovery Orientation of Treatment, Consumer Empowerment, and Satisfaction with Services: a Mediational Model', *Psychiatric Rehabilitation Journal*, XXXIV, 2, 153–6.

Blakemore, K. (2003). *Social Policy: An Introduction. Second Edition* (Open University Press. Buckingham).

Brohan, E., Gauci, D., Sartorius, N., Thornicroft, G. and GAMIAN-Europe Study Group (2011). 'Self-Stigma, Empowerment and Perceived Discrimination among

People with Bipolar Disorder or Depression in 13 European Countries: The GAMIAN–Europe Study', *Journal of Affective Disorders*, CXXIX, 1–3, 56–63.

Crane-Ross, D., Lutz, W. J. and Roth, D. (2006). 'Consumer and Case Manager Perspectives of Service Empowerment: Relationship to Mental Health Recovery', *Journal of Behavioral Health Services & Research*, XXXIII(2), 142–55.

EU COM (2001). 'Communication for the Commission, Making a European Area of Lifelong Learning a Reality' (European Commission, November 2001, Luxembourg). *http://eur-lex.europa.eu/LexUriServ/LexUriServ.do?uri= COM:2001:0678:FIN:EN:PDF*, date accessed 14 June 2011.

Garber, J. and Seligman, M. (1980). *Human Helplessness Theory and Applications* (New York Academic Press).

Jormfeldt, H., Arvidsson, B., Svensson, B. and Hansson, L. (2008). 'Construct Validity of a Health Questionnaire Intended to Measure the Subjective Experience of Health among Patients in Mental Health Services', *Journal of Psychiatric and Mental Health Nursing*, 1XV, 3, 238–45.

Lecomte T., Cyr M., Lesage A. D., Wilde J., Leclerc C. and Ricard N. (1999). 'Efficacy of a Self-Esteem Module in the Empowerment of Individuals with Schizophrenia', *Journal of Nervous and Mental Disease*, CLXXXVII, 406–13.

Nelson, G., Lord, J. and Ochocka, J. (2001). 'Empowerment and Mental Health in the Community: Narratives of Psychiatric and Consumer Survivors', *Journal of Community Applied Social Psychology*, 11(2), 125–42.

Rowlands, J. (1995). 'Empowerment Examined', *Development in Practice*, 5, 101–7.

Ryan, M. and Deci, E. (2000). 'Self Determination Theory and the Facilitation of Intrinsic Motivation, Social Development and Well-Being', *American Psychologist*, LV, 68–78.

Sibitz, I., Amering, M., Unger, A., Seyringer, M. E., Bachmann, A., Schrank, B., Benesch, T., Schulze, B. and Woppmann, A. (2011). 'The Impact of the Social Network, Stigma and Empowerment on the Quality of Life in Patients with Schizophrenia', *European Psychiatry*, XXVI, 1, 28–33.

Silver, M., Conte, R., Miceli, M. and Poggi, I. (1986). 'Humiliation: Feeling, Social Control and the Construction of Identity', *Journal for the Theory of Social Behaviour*, XVI, 269–83.

Syme, L. (1988). 'Social Epidemiology and the Work Environment International', *Journal of Health Services*, XVIII, 635–45.

Thompson, S. and Spacapan, S. (1991). 'Perceptions of Control in Vulnerable Populations', *Journal of Social Issues*, XLVII, 1–21.

Trainor, J. and Tremblay, J. (1992). 'Consumer/Survivor Businesses in Ontario: Challenging the Rehabilitation Model', *Canadian Journal of Community Mental Health*, XI(2), 65–71.

Tyers, C. and Aston, J. (2002). 'Impact of the Adult and Community Learning Fund', *Institute for Employment Studies*. (Brighton, UK), *http://archive.niace.org.uk/funds/ ACLF/ACLF_Impact_Study_Final_Report.pdf*, date accessed 15 December 2011.

United Nations (2006). *Convention on the Rights of Persons with Disabilities and its Optional Protocol* (New York), http://www.un.org/disabilities/default. asp?id=150, date accessed 14 June 2011.

United Nations Development Report (1995). Human Development Report (New York: Oxford University Press).

Vauth, R., Kleim, B., Wirtz, M. and Corrigan, P. W. (2007). 'Self-Efficacy and Empowerment as Outcomes of Self-Stigmatizing and Coping in Schizophrenia', *Psychiatry Research*, CL (1), 71–80.

Wallerstein, N. (2006). 'What is the Evidence on Effectiveness of Empowerment to Improve Health?' (Copenhagen, WHO Regional Office for Europe), Health Evidence Network report; http://www.euro.who.int/Document/E88086.pdf, date accessed June 2011.

Ware, N. (1999). 'Evolving Consumer Households: An Experiment in Community Living for People with People with Severe Psychiatric Disorders', *Psychiatric Rehabilitation Journal*, XXIII, 3–10.

World Health Organization (1986). 'Ottawa Charter for Health Promotion', http://www.who.int/hpr/NPH/.../ottawa_charter_hp.pdf, date accessed 14 October 2010.

World Health Organization (2005). 'Bangkok Charter for Health Promotion in a Globalized World', http://www.who.int/healthpromotion/conferences/6gchp/bangkok_charter/en/index.html, date accessed 14 October 2010.

WHO Regional Office for Europe (2005a). 'Mental Health Declaration for Europe'. Copenhagen, WHO Regional Office for Europe, http://www.euro.who.int/en/what-we-do/health-topics/diseases-and-conditions/mental-health/policy, date accessed 15 June 2010.

WHO Regional Office for Europe (2009). 'Policies and Practices for Mental Health in Europe – Meeting the Challenges'. WHO Regional Office for Europe, Copenhagen.

10
Evaluating Service-User Involvement in Mental Health Services

David Crepaz-Keay

Service-user involvement: my own story

If service-user involvement is to continue to change lives, to continue to inspire, to make a difference, we need to be able to demonstrate its worth, to measure its impact, to prove its effectiveness. I started life as an economist and statistician. Had I not gone mad at an early age, I may well still be an economist or statistician. I spent my formative years almost equally divided between a traditional English education and being a traditional English mental patient. These parallel lives felt very different to me: half my life was spent learning, growing and becoming respected for my knowledge and skills: by the time I left university I had a degree in economics and statistics and had written models of government debt interest for the Treasury; by the time I left psychiatric hospital, I had six psychiatric diagnoses finally settling on schizophrenia, over a dozen different treatments, and had been told not to expect too much from life. The company was different as well: economists were almost entirely a white middle class group, mental patients were not. But the biggest difference was the attitude of other people: in those days, economists were treated with respect, and even deference; mental patients in general, and schizophrenics in particular, were society's untouchables.

It was years of flipping between these two completely different existences that drove me into service-user involvement. I could not understand, I still cannot understand, how the same person, me, could be treated so differently just because of the way I was introduced to people. This was simple discrimination. We now know (though it has been fairly apparent for years) that one of the most effective ways to challenge discrimination is to expose the discriminators to the objects of their discrimination in a positive context. We also know that some of the most significant discrimination comes from medical people in general and psychiatric staff in particular. This is not as odd as you might think: during my divided life, psychiatric staff only saw me at my most mad, they never saw the economist within, whereas my treasury colleagues saw the lot, for better or worse, and made up their own minds about the whole me.

Getting involved in user involvement was the most important step I took. I remember the first time I met other mad people, talking about their madness as a part of them – not as some alien growth that needed treatment or removal. I remember the excitement felt when I first spoke in public about my experiences and people listened without trying to diagnose or treat me. I have been involved in involvement since the 1980s, a world unrecognisable today. Now, the language of involvement and empowerment is everywhere. What I say now is no longer seen as radical or mad. What used to be seen as heretical (for example, proposing that patients could be part of the process of recruiting staff) is now part of contract specification or service level agreement.

Making involvement effective

Service-user involvement is important, but it needs to be effective, it needs to make a difference to people's lives. I have seen service-user involvement in many services across Britain and there are a number of things that the most effective involvement approaches have in common. In order to ensure its effectiveness, it is useful to be able to measure the impact of service-user involvement. Although this is neither common practice, nor indeed straightforward, it becomes increasingly difficult to promote service-user involvement without paying attention to its costs and benefits. However, before identifying ways of measuring effective service-user involvement, it is worth setting out some basic foundations for effective service-user involvement so that we can build on these to measure involvement.

1. *Be clear about the purpose of service-user involvement*
   Service-user involvement is more likely to be successful if you think clearly about why you are doing it. This applies equally to service providers and service users. If the purpose is not clear or if service users are not clear why they are getting involved and what they want out of involvement, then it is likely to be doomed from the start. If, on the other hand, everyone knows why they are there and what they want then chances of success are considerably greater.

2. *Be clear about the limits of involvement*

When setting out to involve users in service organisation and provision, they need to know what can and what cannot be changed. Many a well-meaning event has turned sour because service users wanted to discuss service opening times and locations while providers wanted to talk about staff recruitment and training (or vice versa). If certain things cannot be changed, say so and everyone can concentrate on those things that might be able to be done differently.

3. *Communicate clearly and regularly*

Service-user involvement is likely to generate both ideas and enthusiasm, but these are precious and delicate and need to be nurtured. There is little worse than getting involved and then thinking you have been forgotten. Not every service-user idea is going to happen at once, some will not happen at all; but if the people responsible for the service-user involvement plan keep everyone involved up to date with what has happened, is happening, will happen and will not happen (and why), then most people will think their involvement has been and will continue to be worthwhile.

Although these factors do not, in themselves, guarantee effective service-user involvement, it is hard to achieve in their absence. It is also important to explore service-user involvement in more detail. For purposes of measuring effective service-user involvement, it is useful to break down involvement into three strata or levels of involvement: individual, organisational and strategic. This is not the only way to analyse involvement, but it works well in most settings

Involvement at a strategic level

Involving people in what tomorrow's services will look like is where service-user involvement really started. Discontent with existing services along with increasing concerns at the widespread abuse of human rights, combined with a move towards greater consumerism in public services in general and health services in particular, gave rise to the idea of involving mental health service users as consumers. Involvement in planning groups and involvement in policy work is widespread in the UK and many other countries. Many service users began involvement at this level. The main advantage of this sort of involvement is that it offers the opportunity for future services to be shaped by people's direct experience of using them. It also exposes policy makers and decision makers to direct contact with service users in expert roles and helps to reduce stereotypes of service users as dependent or incapable. The disadvantage of involvement at this level is that it can be very exclusive, involving small numbers of service users, often from a very narrow cross section of society; it can also be very demanding on those involved and can lead to them feeling isolated from their peers. Service users involved at this level are often criticised for not being truly representative of all service users.

Involvement at and organisational/operational level

Getting involved in the daily running of services is what most people think of when they talk about service-user involvement. This will include everything from involvement in recruiting and training staff to service users running their own services. There are many advantages of involvement at this level, including: the opportunity to directly improve services on the basis of how they are experienced; the chance to involve more people than is possible at a strategic level; the chance to expose frontline staff to the abilities of service users rather than focusing on their disabilities; and the opportunity for service users to develop useful skills. This also has its disadvantages: it may divide service users into those that are seen as capable and those that are seen as incapable, services users may even do this to themselves and their peers; some staff may feel insecure or disempowered by the involvement of service users and some are uneasy about blurring boundaries or eroding professional expertise.

Involvement at an individual level

Involving service users more directly in their own care and treatment and, indeed, giving us more control over our lives is fundamental to all service-user involvement. It is, however, in many ways the least developed level. Most services have been developed as mechanisms to deliver treatment to patients: service users are passive recipients of treatments developed, selected, delivered and evaluated by professional experts. Involvement at the individual level challenges this historical underpinning of our services, professions and indeed the mental health sector as a whole. It is however entirely consistent with emerging rights frameworks both at a European and United Nations level. The advantages of involving people at an individual level are: it works for almost anyone, with people just getting involved as much as possible; it builds confidence; people take more responsibility for their own mental health and are likely to develop more constructive relationships with clinicians and other staff by reaching a common understanding of the benefits and costs of different treatment options. Although this remains the least developed level, there have been a number of developments in recent years that offer potential to significantly increase this most important level of involvement; including the rise of 'personalisation' and increased interest in peer support and self-management.

Once we have outlined the levels at which service-user involvement can occur, and some of the characteristics of good involvement, it becomes easier to assess and measure effective involvement. One of the best ways to identify effective involvement is to look carefully at the people involved. If they are a plentiful and diverse group that reflect the people using or needing a service, it is likely that the involvement is effective. The easiest way to increase the diversity of involvement is to ensure that there is range of mechanisms available for involvement.

To many people organising involvement, involvement means meetings. Most people would rather not spend their time in meetings and most service users are just like most people in this respect; and yet involvement seems obsessed with meetings. They are, however, only one possible mechanism and involvement deserves better. Effective involvement will not avoid meetings altogether, but it will offer people alternatives. Blogs, social networks and online surveys form a significant part of many people's lives today. They offer the potential to involve more people in more ways than could have been imagined twenty years ago; but they rely on skills, resources and access that are often denied to people within psychiatric services. They are, like many predominantly technological advances, also biased towards younger people. This is not a bad thing in itself: involving younger people is a particular challenge and anything which improves involvement amongst younger people and young adults in their twenties should be welcomed.

Technology also offers mechanisms to involve older people, as well as people who may have more limited mobility or capacity. Recent work with graphics, touchscreens and even touch sensitive mats has enabled people to express views, preferences, and even make treatment decisions with the blink of an eye. There are no longer good technical reasons for failing to involve anyone; the most significant barrier remains the lack of will to do it. This takes us firmly back to the importance of being clear about the purpose of involvement.

Table 10.1 above describes different levels of indicators for effective involvement using the framework we have identified, with criteria that

Table 10.1 Service-user involvement indicators

	Who	How	Why
Personal	More people and greater diversity is better	Ensure a good range of mechanisms	Ensure clarity of purpose
Operational	Check for bias to or against particular groups (for example: age, gender, race, diagnosis)	Be aware of things that block particular groups or individuals	Ensure everyone involved understands purpose and limits
Strategic	Ensure this is not the preserve of an elite	Diversity in approaches leads to diversity in involvement	Link involvement initiatives to observable outcomes

should help to assess involvement, enable benchmarking and identify improvement plans.

Good indicators should be generated locally and their generation should be led by service users.

In the framework of the WHO-EC partnership project (WHO Europe 2010) the following (provisional) 19 indicators have been identified:

Protection of Human Rights

- people using mental health services* have the right to vote.
- people using mental health services* have the right to hold public office.
- the country has employment legislation that forbids discrimination in employment on the basis of diagnosis or history of mental illness.
- the country has employment legislation to cover the needs of family carers.

Inclusion in decision-making

- mental health service users and their families are involved in the development of mental health policy and legislation.

* People who either in the past have used or are presently using mental health services.

- mental health service users and their families have authority in the process of designing, planning and implementing mental health services.

High-quality care and accountability of services

- people with mental health problems and their families have access to appropriate mental health services.
- people with mental health problems have access to general health services like other citizens.
- people with mental health problems have the opportunity to be actively involved in the planning and review of their own care.
- families of people with mental health problems have the opportunity to be actively involved in the planning and review of care.
- mental health service users and their families are involved in inspection and monitoring of mental health services.
- people with mental health problems and their families are involved in education and training of staff working in mental health services.

Access to information and resources

- mental health service users have a right to access their medical records.
- people subjected to formal interventions due to their mental health problems have access to affordable legal support.
- people with a disability caused by a mental health problem and their families have equitable access to state benefits.
- public funds are available for national user and family organisations.
- accessible and appropriate information and education about services and treatment is available for people with mental health problems.
- adequate information and education is available for families of people with mental health problems to support them in their role as family carers.
- the welfare benefit system compensates for the financial implications of being a family carer.

A good suite of indicators will help anyone serious about involvement reflect on their own practice and identify improvements for their work. It should also allow those responsible for funding to understand what they get for their money and provide those tasked with regulating or monitoring services with a tool to support their inspections.

Expertise and experience are NOT the same thing. But with support, and a methodical approach, experience can be transformed into expertise. With enough high quality effective involvement, services can be transformed into a powerful tool for positive mental health.

Reference

WHO Regional Office for Europe (2010). 'Empowerment in Mental Health', Statement by the World Health Organization Regional Office for Europe.

11
Lifelong Learning, Mental Health and Higher Education: a UK Focus

Jill Anderson and Janet Holmshaw

Introduction

The growing involvement of people on the receiving end of services in the planning and delivery of care has been accompanied by their engagement, within higher education institutions, in the education of future professionals. Such involvement provides one means by which awareness of lifelong learning and its links with mental health can be developed in those who will become practitioners. It also provides lifelong learning opportunities for those who engage in teaching and research – which may or may not be bolstered by formal training. As a result, service user and carer educators not only teach *about* lifelong learning and its links with empowerment and recovery but *embody* this process. In this chapter, we explore these themes and identify key challenges and opportunities.

Lifelong learning, mental health and higher education: exploring the links

Mental health and higher education

Mental health, as a field, spans a range of professional disciplines in higher education including, but not confined to, social work, nursing, psychology, occupational therapy, and medicine. In the United Kingdom, changes in mental health policy, the introduction of new roles and ways of working, have led to calls for an increased focus in pre- and post-qualifying curricula on social inclusion, empowerment and recovery (DOH 2004), supported by interdisciplinary learning and teaching initiatives such as the Mental Health in Higher Education project (Anderson and Burgess 2007) and the work of the Centres for Excellence in Teaching and Learning about mental health (CEIMH 2011; CETL Mental Health and Social Work 2011). Recent mental health policy (DOH 2009) highlights prevention, public mental health and universal services, with implications for curricula across a range of other disciplines and subject areas: from town planning to librarianship, from sports science to performing arts.

There has, moreover, been a growing awareness – across all disciplines – of the mental wellbeing of both students (Stanley and Manthorpe 2002, RCP 2003) and lecturers (Kinman and Jones 2003), with implications for curriculum development (Burgess, Anderson and Westerby 2009). This has, in part, been prompted by the requirements of the Disability Discrimination Act (1995, 2005) and the Disability Equality Duty which came into force in 2006. Impending change within the higher educa-tion sector is likely to increase rather than to dissipate such concerns. At an institutional level, wellbeing has been identified as a key indica-tor of quality (New Economics Foundation 2008), and the recent public health white paper (DOH 2010) makes explicit mention of the need to promote 'healthy universities'. Mental health and wellbeing is, then, a key – and increasingly debated – concern within a higher education context. We are still at an early stage in translating that awareness into action.

Service-user involvement in teaching and research

The above has been both a trigger for, and in some aspects a result of, the increasing involvement of mental health service users and carers in teaching and research. There is a growing expectation that those with direct lived experience of mental ill-health will contribute to teach-ing in health and social care, though the awareness that there might be learning too to gain from those who have not made formal use of services has been slower to take hold (Gupta and Blewett 2008). The Quality Assurance Agency requires the providers of healthcare educa-tion to involve service users (Skills for Health 2008). Professional bodies are increasingly mandating service-user and carer involvement (GSCC 2002, DOH 2006, Royal College of Psychiatrists 2008, BPS 2008) and, in the case of the General Social Care Council, financially supporting it. An infrastructure has been developing with initiatives such as Social Work Education Participation (SWEP 2011), funded by the Department of Health to develop a network for service user and carer educators involved in the education of social workers.

Service-user involvement in teaching encompasses an ever expanding range of activities. Service users and carers are involved in the recruitment and selection of students, in curriculum development, in the development and delivery of teaching, in assessing students' work or their preparedness for practice, as well as in pedagogical research and evaluation. They are employed in a variety of capacities – as freelance consultants and in visiting lecturer roles.

A number of universities have created service-user and carer involvement posts to support this increasingly complex community engagement work (Ward and Rhodes 2010, Anghel and Ramon 2009). This has resulted, in the case of the Comensus project at the University of Central Lancashire (Comensus 2011), in the organisation of a number of international conferences and a collaboratively written publication (McKeown et al. 2010). Supported by the Mental Health in Higher Education project, the Developers of User and Carer Involvement in Education (DUCIE) network has evolved (DUCIE 2011), providing a support network for user and carer involvement workers employed in UK higher education institutions (Anderson and Burgess 2007). An award scheme for user and carer involvement workers – The Ian Light Award for Work in Pairs – has been developed to acknowledge this increasingly embedded area of practice (mhhe 2011). Moreover, a body of knowledge is developing – encoded in a range of good practice documents (Tew, Gell and Foster 2004, Levin 2004, Essen et al. 2009). Although stigma and discrimination are still rife, in universities as elsewhere in our society, a number of mainstream academics are now open about their own service use (Jamison 1997, Benjamin 2005, Brandon 1997).

Within a research context too, people with lived experience are developing the knowledge base for mental health. There have been a growing number of service-user-led studies (Beresford 2005, Rose 2003, Fox 2007) and a considerable body of expertise has developed to be shared (Wallcraft, Schrank and Amering 2009). Service users are increasingly engaged as co-researchers with academic partners. This creates rich opportunities for the development of knowledge and skills in research on the part of the person with lived experience of mental ill health. It can bring immeasurable benefits too to the academic researcher, and ultimately the consumer of the research – resulting in high quality projects that are grounded in lived experience. A number of examples have been written up (Ramon 2003, Tickle 2009) and others can be accessed on the websites of organisations such as Involve (2011) and Shaping Our Lives (2011).

One might assume that service-user involvement in teaching and in research would be part of a single drive to place lived experience more centrally within development of the knowledge base for health and social care, yet these endeavours can proceed as parallel strands of activity within a single institution. This could be seen as a reflection of the separation of teaching and research activity within the sector as a whole. One might also assume that all of the above activity would link with lifelong learning and widening participation approaches within higher education – those which promote access for people from under-privileged groups. It is to that issue that we now turn.

Lifelong learning and mental health

There are very clear links between learning and mental health – they can interact both positively (Field 2009) and negatively, as recent work on 'troublesome' knowledge highlights (Meyer and Land 2003). There are important examples of public health bodies that acknowledge the role of learning in improving health outcomes, including mental health outcomes. Yet, almost invariably, the focus has been primarily on children and young people – for example, with the promotion of the Social and Emotional Aspects of Learning programme in schools (SEAL). As a result, debate is opening up about the learning that initial teacher trainees should be doing in the area of mental health (Rothi and Leavey 2008); what has been less explored is how the importance of learning itself – and its place in recovery – should feature within the curricula for trainee mental health workers. The only mention of learning in the Ten Essential Shared Capabilities (DOH 2004) – a highly influential UK policy framework providing a user-led definition of the core skills of what should constitute the essential elements of a good quality service – is in relation to workers, rather than those whom they set out to support. Students, while themselves engaged on pro-grammes, may not be encouraged to think about the role of learning in the lives of others.

Yet there is evidence that lifelong learning opportunities are valued by service users (Wertheimer 1997, Ramon et al. 2011).

A range of opportunities are available through mainstream mental health services and, as we shall see below, opportunities are develop-ing in a higher education context too. The Mental Health Partnership Programme, led by the National Institute of Adult Continuing Education (NIACE) in partnership with the Learning and Skills Council and the Inclusion Institute, has sought to influence policy and to support the development of good practice that promotes and improves learning and skills opportunities for people who experience mental health problems. A whole range of resources, developed by this programme are available online (NIACE 2011).

Lifelong learning and higher education

Universities have long been engaged with the lifelong learning agenda. The recent emphases on widening participation, on public engagement and knowledge transfer initiatives are increasing the involvement in higher education of a range of previously underrepresented groups. The National Coordinating Centre for Public Engagement in higher education has recently been established (NCPE 2011) and a Manifesto for Public Engagement has been launched (NCPE 2010). Yet few links have to date been established between the initiatives outlined above and widening participation, knowledge transfer and lifelong learning initiatives. Moreover, despite the rhetoric of support, there has been some curtailment of lifelong learning opportunities (with cuts to summer school programmes for example and to other outreach activities in some institutions). The definition of lifelong learning used within universities can be rather narrow, yet there are those based within the lifelong learning sector who are thinking broadly about the links between lifelong learning and wellbeing (Field 2009).

Our interest in this chapter is in the intersections between lifelong learning, mental health and higher education. The engagement of service users and carers in teaching about mental health within universities is opening up a two way learning process. On the one hand it is providing opportunities for students to learn about recovery, lifelong learning and the links with mental health (as a content area of curricula). On the other hand, it is creating lifelong learning and recovery opportunities for service users. In what follows, we give some examples of those opportunities, returning then to an examination of the wider context – its barriers and challenges as well as the opportunities to be grasped.

Lifelong learning, recovery and the mental health curriculum

There is increasing emphasis in training for mental health professionals on recovery, empowerment and service-user and carer perspectives. Students in higher education, because of their own engagement with learning processes, should be well placed to explore the links between learning and mental wellbeing. However, they may not be helped, on all programmes, to reflect upon how these issues interrelate – either for themselves or for users of mental health services. Service user educators can help students to recognise the intertwined nature of recovery and lifelong learning in a number of ways, as discussed below.

Lifelong learning and recovery as a curriculum content area

The links between lifelong learning and recovery can be articulated by service users through their direct involvement in teaching. This may be explicit when the focus of the teaching session is people's own experiences of recovery and the factors that have helped or hindered this. For example, in reporting the outcome of the initial development of the Psychosis Revisited workshops, Hayward (2004) describes a training intervention where two service users were interviewed by a service user interviewer in front of workshop participants made up of community mental health team and assertive outreach team members. He notes that the focus on recovery in these interviews was important as 'each service user spoke of building lives that were of a better quality, albeit amid the occasional setback, than the lives that had preceded the onset of their psychotic experiences' (Hayward 2004).

In an earlier example, Chapman (1996) discusses an informal teaching setting, a 'dinner conversation', where service users are paired with student nurses and asked to talk about their 'experiences and coping strategies over a crisis'. Similarly, Crosby et al (2009) describe a teaching intervention focused directly upon recovery, where mental health nursing students are split into small discussion groups, each facilitated by two service user educators. The three hour session consists of two parts. It starts with a general discussion of different experiences, perspectives and meanings of recovery. In the second half, participants and educators explore together the ways in which mental health practitioners, especially nurses, can develop their practice to be more recovery orientated.

As well as direct teaching, the development of teaching materials focused upon people's own experiences of recovery can help to promote an understanding of the role of lifelong learning in recovery. The Centre of Excellence in Interdisciplinary Mental Health (CEIMH) at Birmingham University has commissioned and supported the development of video recordings and digital stories made by service users – available as teaching and learning resources on the Centre's website (CEIMH 2011). Online modules on recovery have been developed as part of the Ten Essential Shared Capabilities learning materials (NHS Education for Scotland 2007, CCAWI 2011).

Students have found the input of service users and carers helpful in providing an insight into recovery experience (Hayward 2004, Simpson and Reynolds 2008). For example: 'The most helpful aspect about having service user trainers was explaining their recovery and how they coped with their illness'. (Crosby et al 2009). Arguably, university staff are also learning from the involvement of service users. Tew, Gell and Foster (2004) outline the 'payoffs' for teaching staff in terms of increased job satisfaction and professional development, updated knowledge about mental health and new ideas. Service user and carer colleagues may offer professional and personal support in a way that is different from other colleagues. Staff involved with the Comensus project suggest that involvement with service user and carer educators can provide job fulfilment and a catalyst for reconnection with their professional values. Staff also reported becoming better at relationships with learners, behaving more inclusively in meetings and functioning better in other areas of work, for example writing and research (McKeown et al. 2010). The subjective nature of the user input with its focus on personal experiences makes this a powerful learning experience for students but there is potential for a wider impact too.

Implicit in accounts of the benefits of user and carer involvement in education are the links between lifelong learning and recovery, but it is not obvious the extent to which students are made aware of these. Should lifelong learning experiences form a more explicit content area for curricula?

Service users and carers embodying lifelong learning and recovery

As well as delivering input on these issues, service user educators can influence student learning through their *embodiment* of lifelong learning and recovery, helping students to see that both are possible. Livingstone and Cooper (2004) make the point that, for the most part, mental health professionals spend a lot of their training in hospital settings with people with acute mental health conditions and that this can lead them to develop a pessimistic view of mental health, what the authors have termed 'therapeutic nihilism'. The involvement of service user educators can help to mitigate this. This was one of the points noted by student nurses in their evaluation of the service user led discussions sessions at Middlesex University: 'The realisation that being mentally ill need not be a life sentence provides evidence that recovery is not only possible, but health promotion is integral to this' (Crosby et al. 2009). This can be an especially powerful experience for people working in acute mental health settings. Obi-Udeaja et al. (2010) describe, in a course on the Therapeutic Management of Violence and Aggression, the impact on students of service user educators with experiences of being restrained in mental health settings.

Service user educators learn actively through involvement in mental health training and education, building confidence and self-esteem

(Cole 1994, Frisby 2001, Hayward 2004, Vandrevala 2007) and developing new skills (Masters et al. 2002, Forrest et al. 2000, McKeown et al. 2010). Involvement in direct teaching activities can develop abilities in communication, presentation and the facilitation of teaching and learning activities – for example, through group work and seminar approaches.

There are also examples of more specific skills development. For example, Simpson and Reynolds (2008) describe an e-learning initiative for mental health student nurses in which they took part in online discussion groups with service users from local day centres. One of the many benefits reported by the service users was gaining confidence in using computers. Service user educators have also increased their knowledge and skills in using computer and other technology through developing digital stories as teaching resources with the CEIMH at Birmingham University (Smojkis and Clark 2009).

Involvement can enhance the process of recovery (Masters et al. 2002). One of the findings from the evaluation of the Comensus project is that, although service users first became involved as a way of making a difference to health and social care education, they also discovered that this had beneficial effects for themselves – not only in learning practical skills but also confidence and assertiveness: 'People are moving forward in their lives by helping other people' (McKeown et al. 2010). One of the service users involved in the Psychosis Revisited workshops reflected on this:

> I knew that I needed to open the can of worms and start dealing with the issues that surrounded my traumatic admission to mental health hospital several years ago. I felt that sharing my experiences would help me face them, deal with the feelings and enable me to move forwards.
> (Hayward 2004)

A service user educator from the Therapeutic Management of Violence and Aggression training described the experience as both cathartic and enabling:

> The reason I like teaching is that it gives me time to bring out a lot of things that I have inside, good or bad
> (Obi-Udeaja et al. 2010, p. 189).

The learning processes that service user and carer educators are engaged in can be made visible to students. It may also be possible for students to recognise the links between lifelong learning and mental health and wellbeing through reflection on their *own* experiences. Service user educators may have a role to play in this within a higher education setting, counteracting what has been described as an 'emotion-free zone' (Leathwood and Hey 2009) and enabling students to reflect on their own wellbeing as they make their journey through a programme. Tew, Gell and Foster (2004, p. 14) make the point that the 'explicit involvement of users and carers in education can pave the way for students and teaching staff to be more open about their own experiences – and for these experiences to be valued and used as a resources within the learning process'.

There are increasing examples of service users taking on mentoring support roles with students: the 'Buddy scheme' in Kent, for example, where nursing and midwifery students are mentored in their practice placements by a mental health service user 'buddy' (Buddy scheme 2010). A joint project between Surrey and Canterbury Christ Church Universities paired service users as placement advisors to trainee clinical psychologists and found that this had a significant influence on trainees' learning and practice (Hayward and Cooke 2008).

Collaborative learning initiatives

Finally, service user educators can help students to make links between lifelong learning, recovery and empowerment through engaging with them as co-learners. This is more than modelling lifelong learning; it is learning in partnership. Rowley (2000) reports an innovative way of involving service users within training programmes as course members alongside social services staff – on mental health training courses for community care staff. McAndrew and Samociuk (2003) describe setting up a group of service users and students within the mental health nurse training to reflect upon and discuss mental health issues. Tee and Coldham (2004) present a cooperative enquiry-based initiative involving mental health nursing students and service users.

Another example of collaborative learning, this time including academics, is given by Lefroy and Hutton (2009). Their initial project was to develop a training programme for service users and carers to help prepare them for participation and involvement. However, this was expanded in recognition that it was not just the users and carer participants who needed such an induction. As a result of this, a half-day 'What is Participation' training session was developed for all involved in their BA Social Work programme: practitioners, lecturers, students and service users and carers.

Similarly, mental health practitioners and service users learn together on the Short Course in Classroom Teaching at Middlesex University. This course is designed for health and social care practitioners and service user and carer educators who are involved in training and teaching on the Mental Health and Social Work programmes at Middlesex University, or similar programmes, or who may wish to develop knowledge, skills, experience and confidence in these areas in order to become involved at a later date (CETL Mental Health and Social Work 2011).

Creating formal lifelong learning opportunities for users and carers in higher education settings

Service user and carer educators can learn through active engagement in teaching, as above. More formal opportunities may also be provided.

Learning about involvement

In many of the initiatives mentioned above, some form of structured training and support is provided for the service user and carer educators. In 'Learning from Experience', a guide to good practice in involving service users and carers in mental health education, Tew, Gell and Foster (2004) include a number of examples of such training initiatives throughout the country. For example, to help prepare service users to teach mental health nursing students, training based upon a teaching and assessment module for nurses was delivered (Hanson and Mitchell 2001). Sometimes more specialised training is provided. For example, on the MA in Community Mental Health at Birmingham University, service user educators involved in assessing students' written work were given training on providing feedback (Bailey 2005).

In some cases the universities themselves provide the training (Hansen and Mitchell 2001, Lefroy and Hutton 2009, Simpson and Reynolds 2008); in others, this has been delivered by local service user groups: CEIMH has supported Birmingham Mind to develop and provide a train the trainers programme (CEIMH 2009), and presentation skills training for the Comensus service user and carer engagement project was commissioned from a local service user led training group (McKeown et al. 2010).

There are also examples of training courses offering participants university credits if they wish to complete an assessed element of the programme, for example the short course in classroom teaching at Middlesex University (mentioned above). Similarly, there are increasing examples of training courses delivered by external organisations also offering accreditation for those who wish to carry out course assignments: Mind in Harrow, Together and Education Not Discrimination (part of the Time to Change initiative) have accredited their 'train the trainers' programmes with Middlesex University.

Providing training, and support to service user educators is seen not only as a way of improving the quality of the teaching experience but also of providing opportunities for the service user educators to develop skills that can be used in work related roles or employment (Bailey 2005). Tew, Gell and Foster (2004) make the point that involvement in mental health education may provide a starting point for employment in educational settings or mental health services – or in the broader world of work.

Learning in other areas

There are other kinds of lifelong learning programmes for service users being set up within universities, unrelated to training or research. Two examples are: the Experienced Involvement project, an 'Experts by Experience' qualification funded by the European Commission's Leonardo Da Vinci Programme, the aim of which is to 'springboard service users into mental health employment' (EX-IN 2010); and the Leadership and Empowerment in Mental Health course at Liverpool John Moores University aimed at providing learning and development opportunities for mental health service users who wish to get involved in consultation work (LJMU 2011).

Moreover, mainstream mental health services are beginning to migrate to educational settings. The Recovery Education Program at the Center for Psychiatric Rehabilitation at Boston University in the US, for example, is aimed at those who are 'willing to use an educational environment to foster their recovery' (Boston Center for Psychiatric Rehabilitation 2011). It is an adult education programme, open to individuals with a documented diagnosis of a psychiatric illness, that offers students the opportunity to choose a range of wellness courses that support their treatment, rehabilitation and recovery. The Centre also offers the Training for the Future programme – an intensive one-year vocational recovery programme for people who wish to pursue a career and need computer and work readiness skills. Students attend classes four full days a week for one semester while learning typing, Microsoft Word, Excel, Access, PowerPoint, and some website design. They also participate in recovery seminars and wellness courses. A supported education programme is a further aspect of the centre's work.

Initiatives based in Higher Education go beyond mental health into other areas: '*Storying Sheffield*' is a unique venture in British higher education. Half of the participants are second-year undergraduates (known as 'long-course students') studying for a degree in English Literature. The rest of the participants are people from the city who come from groups which have tended to be socially excluded ('short-course students'). For the first year of the course, most short-course students are long-term users of mental health services. Short course students hold University student status, and have access to all University facilities and resources' (Storying Sheffield 2011). *Out of Character* is a theatre company comprised of people who use mental health services and staff and students at York St John University. The company has a particular interest in developing educational and theatre-based opportunities with people who use mental health services (Out of Character 2010). The company has grown out of courses in theatre taught by tutors and students on the undergraduate theatre programme and offered to people who use mental health services.

Looking to the future

Higher education institutions can, without a doubt, provide fertile ground for connections between lived experience of mental ill health and lifelong learning – providing opportunities for mental health service users to engage in both teaching and learning and embedding notions of lifelong learning in the education of future health and social care practitioners. Whether that occurs is, of course, partly down to the individuals involved and the ways in which such learning opportunities are developed and facilitated. Some aspects of involvement require particular thought and working through. An analysis of the potential pitfalls of involvement is beyond the scope of this chapter but is beginning to be addressed in the literature (Stickley 2010).

The higher education *context* does provide particular challenges though, and those we will examine briefly here. There are potential barriers to future progress and, indeed, evidence from some quarters that things may be starting to move backwards.

Barriers in the higher education setting

Barriers to the meaningful involvement of service users and carers within a higher education setting were identified at a Mental Health in Higher Education project workshop, held in Derby in June 2003, summarised by Basset, Campbell and Anderson (2006) and have been expanded upon in more recent publications (McKeown et al. 2010). Although a number of examples of good practice have been highlighted in this chapter, hierarchies can make it difficult for people with experience of mental ill health to gain employment and influence within universities as elsewhere in society.

Moreover, despite widening participation initiatives, the forces of stigma and discrimination may combine to restrict access – to both teaching and learning opportunities – for those with lived experience of mental ill health (McKeown et al. 2010). Although a range of programmes have been opening up to students from a wider diversity of backgrounds, pressure to maintain timely completion rates is likely to result in a reluctance, on the part of admissions tutors, to admit those at high risk of becoming unwell.

While considerable progress has been made in validating and accrediting programmes for mental health service users in some institutions, progress has been patchy across the sector, with limited transfer of learning from one university to another. Moreover, changes to the government's Equivalent or Lower Degree Qualification (ELQ) framework have threatened lifelong learning initiatives within universities (Sperlinger 2009).

Funding cuts

User and carer educators have the potential, as we have seen, to drive forward an understanding of the links between lifelong learning and recovery. It is as yet unclear what the implications will be of the current round of funding cuts. Universities, under pressure to cut back on their teaching budgets, may start to see both service user and carer involvement in teaching, and support for lifelong learning initiatives, as non-essential 'extras'. The dissolution of bodies such as the General Social Care Council and the Higher Education Academy Subject Centres may result in a reduced pot of money to support user and carer involvement initiatives. The end of funding for the Centres of Excellence in Teaching and Learning will also have an impact, as several were active in supporting such developments. There are already a number of institutions that were at the forefront of good practice in involving service users and carers in education that, on the departure of an existing service user and carer development worker, have chosen not to reappoint. Likewise, continuing education units are, in some places, under threat.

Levers and opportunities

The picture is far from bleak however. As will be apparent from the above, the past decade has seen considerable progress in widening participation initiatives, support for lifelong learning and the engagement of service users and carers – as both teachers and learners – within a higher education context. Although there is considerable variation both across disciplines and across the country, there has been a growing awareness of the diversity of links between learning, mental health and recovery and the pivotal role for those with lived experience of mental ill-health in illuminating them.

- New communities of practice including the Developers of User and Career Involvement network (DUCIE), the National Survivor User Network (NSUN), Shaping Our Lives, Advocacy and Social Work Education Participation have evolved to a point where they can offer support to people with lived experience of mental ill health who wish to be involved in higher education, as teachers or as learners. This will help to bolster workers within initiatives which may be struggling to survive.
- Some universities are prioritising this area of work. The Inclusion Institute (2011), for example, is a national and international centre for learning, evidence, innovation and practice on inclusion with the person, in the community, through co-production. It is part of the International School for Communities, Rights and Inclusion (ISCRI) at the University of Central Lancashire (UCLan) and maintains a bridge-building database which includes projects with a focus on education.
- As indicated in the introduction to this chapter, there is a growing awareness of wellbeing agendas within a higher education setting. The New Economics Foundation report (2008) – *University Challenge: a wellbeing approach to quality in higher education* – has emphasised the importance of mental health to the effective functioning of higher education institutions. Links between learning and mental wellbeing, within a higher education context, are beginning to be drawn.

A number of initiatives continue to exist for the sharing of good practice: the Mental Wealth UK project (2011) is drawing together those with an interest in student mental health promotion and prevention; the Wellbeing in Higher Education project (2011) is focusing attention on staff wellbeing issues; the Mental Health in Higher Education project (2011) acts as a hub for the sharing of approaches to learning and teaching about mental health.

Conclusion

On the one hand then, universities are proving fruitful ground for lifelong learning and recovery from mental health problems, and an understanding of their links, to flourish. On the other, there are significant obstacles and barriers. The involvement of service users and carers within higher education institutions, and a growing awareness of mental wellbeing as an issue that affects both teachers and learners, is beginning to shift the paradigm but we may now be entering a period of retrenchment and there are challenges ahead.

If those involved in higher education are to rise to these then there is a need to

- continue to nurture those communities of practice that have evolved over recent years and to build bridges between the service user and carer involvement movement and broader public engagement and lifelong learning initiatives within universities.

- develop links between educators in schools, Further Education colleges, universities and third sector organisations, to foster a holistic understanding of links between learning through the lifecycle and mental health.

- embed an understanding of lifelong learning as an important element of recovery in pre- and post-registration initiatives in health and social care.

- encourage students in those disciplines to reflect on the impact of the learning experiences that they are engaged in for their own mental health.

References

Anderson, J. and Burgess, H. (2007). 'Educators Learning Together: Linking Communities of Practice', in T. Stickley and T. Basset (eds). *Teaching and Learning Mental Health* (Chichester: John Wiley).

Anghel, R. and Ramon, S. (2009). 'Service Users and Carers' Involvement in Social Work Education: Lessons from an English Case Study', *European Journal of Social Work* XII(2): 185–199.

Bailey, D. (2005). 'Using an Action Research Approach to Involving Service Users in the Assessment of Professional Competence'? *European Journal of Social Work* VIII(2) 165–79.

Basset, T., Campbell, P. and Anderson, J. (2006). 'Service User/Survivor Involvement in Education and Training – Overcoming the Barriers', *Social Work Education*XXV 25(4), 393–402.

Beresford, P. (2005). 'Social Approaches to Madness and Distress: User Perspectives and User Knowledges', Ch 2 in J. Tew (ed.). *Social Perspectives in Mental Health* (London: JKP).

Benjamin, A. (2005). 'Out in the Lead', *Guardian*, 5 January, 5, http://www.guardian.co.uk/society/2005/jan/05/mentalhealth.guardiansocietysupplement, date accessed 6 January 2011.

Boston Center for Psychiatric Rehabilitation (2011). Recovery Programme, http://www.bu.edu/cpr/services/health/, date accessed 7 January 2011.

Brandon, D. (1997). 'Life: a Course in Survival', *Times Higher Education*, 14 November, http://www.timeshighereducation.co.uk/story.asp?storyCode=10 4608&sectioncode=26, date accessed 6 January 2011.

British Psychological Society (2008). *Good Practice Guidelines: Service User and Carer Involvement within Clinical Psychology Training* (London: BPS, Division of Clinical Psychology).

'Buddy Scheme' (2010). at Kent and Medway NHS and Social Care Partnership Trust, http://www.thebuddyscheme.co.uk/, date accessed 15 December 2010.

Burgess, H., Anderson, J. and Westerby, N. (2009). *Mental Wellbeing and the Curriculum* (York: Higher Education Academy).

Centre of Excellence in Interdisciplinary Mental Health (CEIMH 2011). www.bham.ac.uk/ceimh, date accessed 7 January 2011.

Centre for Clinical and Academic Workforce Innovation (2011). 'Creating and Inspiring Hope – Recovery', http://visit.lincoln.ac.uk/C6/C12/CCAWI/ESC%20Recovery/Forms/AllItems.aspx, date accessed 7 January 2011.

Centre of Excellence in Teaching and Learning for Mental Health and Social Work (2011). http://www.mdx.ac.uk/aboutus/Schools/hssc/mh-sw/cetl/index.aspx, date accessed 7 January 2011.

Chapman, V. (1996). 'Consumers as Faculty: Experts in their Own Lives', *Journal of Psychosocial Nursing and Mental Health Services*, XXXIV, 47–9.

Cole, A. (1994). 'It was an Education: Service Users Assess Student Social Workers', *Community Living*, January 16–17.

Com (2001). 'Employment, Economic Reforms and Social Cohesion – towards a Europe based on innovation and knowledge', The EU Lisbon Summit 23–24 March 2000, (European Commission Luxembourg).

Com (2003). 'Implementing Lifelong Learning Strategies in Europe' [EU and EFTA/EEA countries], Progress report on the follow-up to the Council resolution of 2002 (European Commission Bruxelles 2003).

Com (2009). 'Key Competences for a Changing World'. Draft 2010 joint progress report of the Council and the Commission on the implementation of the 'Education & Training 2010 work programme', Commission of the European Communities Brussels, 25.11.2009, COM(2009) 640 final. SEC (2009) 1598.

Comensus (2011). http://www.uclan.ac.uk/health/schools/school_of_nursing/health_comensus.php, date accessed 9 January 2011.

Crosby, K., Holmshaw, J., Jones, P. and Lynch, C. (2009). 'Service User Involvement in Teaching and Assessment in Student Mental Health Nurse Training', workshop presented at the Showcasing User and Carer Involvement in Education and Practice conference, Birmingham University, 10 November.

Department of Health (DOH) (2004). *The Ten Essential Shared Capabilities: A Framework for the Whole of the Mental Health Workforce*, 40339, (London: Department of Health).

Department of Health (DOH) (2006). *From Values to Action: The Chief Nursing Officer's Review of Mental Health Nursing* (London: HMSO).

Department of Health (DOH) (2009). *New Horizons: A Shared Vision for Mental Health* (London: HMSO).

DUCIE (2011). www.mhhe.heacademy.ac.uk/ducie, date accessed 7 January 2011.

Essen, C., Anderson, J., Clark, M., Cook, J., Edwards, L., Fox, L., Light, I., MacMahon, A., Malihi-Shoja, L., Patel, R., Samociuk, S., Simpson, A., Tang, L. and Westerby, N. (2009). *Involving Service Users and Carers in Education: The Development Worker Role: Guidelines for Higher Education Institutions* (Lancaster, Mental Health in Higher Education), http://www.mhhe.heacademy.ac.uk/ducieguidelines, date accessed 6 January 2011.

EX-IN (2010). Experienced Involvement Project, http://www.ex-in.info/, date accessed 3 January 2011.

Field, J. (2009). 'Good for Your Soul? Adult Learning and Mental Well-Being', *International Journal of Lifelong Education*, XXVIII(2), 175–91.

Forrest, S., Risk, I., Masters, H. and Brown, N. (2000). 'Mental Health Service User Involvement in Nurse Education: Exploring the Issues', *Journal of Psychiatric and Mental Health Nursing*, 7, 51–7.

Fox, J. (2007). 'Experience of Mental Health Recovery and the Service User Researcher', *Ethics and Social Welfare* 1(2), 219–23.

Frisby, R. (2001). 'User Involvement in Mental Health Branch Education: Client Review Presentations', *Nurse Education Today*, XXI, 663–9.

GSCC (2002). *Requirements for Social Work Training* (London: General Social Care Council).

Gupta, A. and Blewett, J. (2008). 'Involving Services Users in Social Work Training on the Reality of Family Poverty: A Case Study of a Collaborative Project', *Social Work Education* XXVII(5): 459–73.

Hanson, B. and Mitchell, D. P. (2001). 'Involving Mental Health Service Users in the Classroom: A Course of Preparation', *Nurse Education in Practice*, I, 120–6.

Hayward, M. (2004). *Service User Involvement in Training: A Catalyst for Collaboration*, a Mental Health in Higher Education Case, http://www.mhhe.heacademy.ac.uk/resources/case-study-13/, date accessed 5 July 2011.

Hayward, M. and Cooke, A. (2008). *Influencing Practice: The Involvement of Service Users and Carers within the Placement Activity of Clinical Psychology Trainees* (Higher Education Academy Psychology Network), http://www.psychology.heacademy.ac.uk/s.php?p=256&db=74, date accessed 3 January 2011.

Inclusion Institute (2011). http://www.uclan.ac.uk/iscri/pmhsi/inclusion_institute.php, date accessed 7 January 2011.

INVOLVE (2011). www. invo.org.uk, date accessed 2 February 2011.

Jamison, K. R. (1997). *An Unquiet Mind* (London: Vintage).

Kinman, G. and Jones, F. (2003). 'Running Up the Down Escalator: Stressors and Strains in UK Academics', *Quality in Higher Education* IX(1), 21–38.

Leathwood, C. and Hey, V. (2009). 'Gender/ed Discourses and Emotional Sub-texts: Theorising Emotion in UK Higher Education', *Teaching in Higher Education*, XIV(4), 429–40.

Lefroy, L. and Hutton, P. (2009). *Getting to Grips with Participation*, Project report of an Ian Light Award http://www.mhhe.heacademy.ac.uk/networks/ian-light-award/getting-to-grips-with-participation/, date accessed 14 June 2011.

Levin, E. (2004). *Involving Service Users and Carers in Social Work Education* (London: Social Care Institute for Excellence).

LJMU (2011). Liverpool John Moores University http://www.ljmu.ac.uk/courses/cpd/75219.htm, date accessed 9 January 2011.

Livingstone, G. and Cooper, C. (2004). 'User and Carer Involvement in Mental Health Training', *Advances in Psychiatric Rehabilitation*, X, 85–92.

Masters, H., Forrest, S., Harley, A., Hunter, M., Brown, N. and Risk, I. (2002). 'Involving Mental Health Service Users and Carers in Curriculum Development: Moving Beyond Classroom Involvement', *Journal of Psychiatric and Mental Health Nursing*, IX, 309–16.

McAndrew, S. and Samociuk, G. A. (2003). 'Reflecting Together: Developing a New Strategy for Continuous User Involvement in Mental Health Nurse Education', *Journal of Psychiatric and Mental Health Nursing*, X(5), 616–21.

McKeown, M., Malihi-Shoja, L., Downe, S. and Supporting the Comensus Writing Collective (2010). *Service User and Carer Involvement in Education for Health and Social Care* (Oxford: Wiley-Blackwell).

Mental Wealth UK (2011). http://www.mentalwealthuk.com/, date accessed 7 January 2011.

Meyer, J. H. F. and Land, R. (2003). 'Threshold Concepts and Troublesome Knowledge (1): Linkages to Ways of Thinking and Practising within the Disciplines'. Enhancing Teaching-Learning Environments in Undergraduate Courses Project, Occasional Report 4.

mhhe (2011). www.mhhe.heacademy.ac.uk, date accessed 7 January 2011.

National Coordinating Centre for Public Engagement (2011). http://www.publicengagement.ac.uk/, date accessed 7 January 2011.

National Coordinating Centre for Public Engagement (2010). *The Engaged University: A Manifesto for Public Engagement* (Bristol: NCPE).

National Institute for Adult and Continuing Education (2011). Mental Health Partnership Programme http://www.niace.org.uk/current-work/area/mental-health, date accessed 7 January 2011.

New Economics Foundation (2008). *University Challenge: A Wellbeing Approach to Quality in Higher Education* (London: New Economics Foundation). Available: http://www.eauc.org.uk/file_uploads/new_economics_forum_university_challenge.pdf, date accessed 6 January 2011.

NHS Education for Scotland/Scottish Recovery Network (2007). *Realising Recovery: A National Framework for Learning and Training in Recovery Focused Practice* (Edinburgh: NES/SRN), www.nes.scot.nhs.uk/mentalhealth/publications/documents/ date accessed 6 January 2011.

Obi-Udeaja, J., Crosby, K., Ryan, G., Sukhram, D. and Holmshaw, J. (2010). 'Service User Involvement in Training for the Therapeutic Management of Violence and Aggression', *Mental Health and Learning Disability Research and Practice*, VII(2), 185–94.

Ogunleye, J., (2009a). 'Lifelong Learning Provision for Mental Health Service Users: An EMILIA Research Report on Disparities, Similarities and a Common European Social Policy Agenda', in N. Popov, C. Wolhuter, B. Leutwyler and J. Ogunleye (eds). *Teacher Training, Education Policy and Social Inclusion*, VII (Sofia, Bulgaria: Bureau for Educational Services), 281–5.

Ogunleye, J. (2009b), 'What about Europe's 'Other' Adult Learners? A Transnational Comparative Study of Lifelong Learning Provision for People with Long-Term Mental Illness', *Proceedings of the IASK International Conference (Peer Review), Teaching and Learning 2009* (Porto, Portugal).

Out of Character (2010). 'Always Ask Yourself: Have I got enough Compassion?', Workshop presented at the 'Living and Learning, Learning and Teaching: Mental Health in Higher Education Conference', Lancaster University, 30–1 March.

Ramon, S., Griffiths, C., Nieminen, I., Pedersen, M. L. and Dawson, I. (2011). 'Towards Social Inclusion through Lifelong Learning in Mental Health: Analysis of Change in the Lives of the EMILIA Project Service Users', *International Journal of Social Psychiatry*, 57(3), 211–23.

Ramon S. (ed.) (2003). *Users Researching Health and Social Care: An Empowering Agenda?* (Birmingham: Venture Press).

Rose, D. (2003). 'Having a Diagnosis is a Qualification for the Job', *BMJ*, 326(7402), 1331.

Rothi, D. M. and Leavey, G. (2008). 'On the Front-line: Teachers as Active Observers of Pupils' Mental Health', *Teaching and Teacher Education* XXIV(5), 1217–31.

Rowley, D. (2000). 'Tapping into Experience', *Community Care*, 5 June.

Royal College of Psychiatrists (2008). *Fair Deal for Mental Health* (London: RCP).

Royal College of Psychiatrists (2003). *The Mental Health of Students in Higher Education* (London: RCP).

Shaping Our Lives (2011). www.shapingourlives.org.uk, date accessed 2 February 2011.

Simpson, A. and Reynolds, L. (2008), 'Consulting the Experts', *Openmind*, CLII, 18–19.

Skills for Health (2008). *Enhancing Quality in Partnership: Healthcare Education QA Framework* (London: Skills for Health).

Smojkis, M. and Clark, M. (2009). 'Digital Stories: Developing Reusable Learning Objects for Use in Health and Social Care Education', workshop presented at the 'Showcasing User and Carer Involvement in Education and Practice conference', Birmingham University, 10 November.

Social Work Education Participation (2011). http://www.socialworkeducation. org.uk/, date accessed 7 January 2011.

Sperlinger, T. (2009). 'How is Denying People a Life-changing Second Chance in Any Way Fair?', *Times Higher Education*, 2 April.

Stanley, N. and Manthorpe, J. (2002). *Students' Mental Health Needs: Problems and Responses*, (London: Jessica Kingsley Publishers).

Stickley, T., Stacey, G., K. Pollock, G., Smith, A., Betinis, J. and Fairbank, S. (2010). 'The Practice Assessment of Student Nurses by People who use Mental Health Services', *Nurse Education Today*, XXX, (1) 20–5.

Storying Sheffield (2011). http://www.storyingsheffield.com/, date accessed 7 January 2011.

Tee, S. and Coldham, T. (2004). *Students and Service Users Learn Together: Co-operative Enquiry and its Implications for Curriculum Development*, a Mental Health in Higher Education Case, http://www.mhhe.heacademy.ac.uk/resources/-case-study-14/, date accessed 5 July 2011.

Tew, J., Gell, C. and Foster, S. (2004). *Learning from Experience: Involving Service Users and Carers in Mental Health Education* (Higher Education Academy, http:// www.mhhe.heacademy.ac.uk/silo/files/learning-from-experience-whole-guide. pdf, accessed 15 December 2011).

Tickle, L. (2009). 'For Academic Researchers Mental Illness Can be an Advantage', *The Guardian*. 25 August.

Vandrevala, T., Hayward, M., Willis, J. and John, M. (2007). 'A Move Towards a Culture of Involvement: Involving Service Users and Carers in the Selection of Future Clinical Psychologists', *Journal of Mental Health Training, Education and Practice*, II(3) 34–43.

Wallcraft, J., Schrank, B. and Amering, M. (2009). *Handbook of Service User Involvement in Mental Health Research* (Chichester: Wiley-Blackwell).

Ward, L. J. and Rhodes, C. A. (2010). 'Embedding Consumer Culture in Health and Social Care Education – A University Office's Perspective', *International Journal of Consumer Studies*, XXXIV (5), 596–602.

Wellbeing in Higher Education (2011). http://www.wellbeing.ac.uk/ date accessed 7 January 2011.

Wertheimer, A. (1997). *Images of Possibility: Creating Learning Opportunities for Adults with Mental Health Difficulties* (Leicester: NIACE).

12

Lifelong Learning and Well-Being: The Health Benefits of Lifelong Learning for People with Mental Illness

James Ogunleye, Chris Griffiths, Ian Dawson and Klavs Nybjerg

Introduction

This chapter situates lifelong learning and mental health within the broader context of the European Union lifelong learning policy agenda, an agenda that places a significant emphasis on promoting social inclusion of multiple disadvantaged groups such as unemployed people with mental health problem. In this chapter, lifelong learning provision denotes *learning* programmes, courses or training for people with mental illness (henceforth referred to as mental health service users or service users for short). The chapter draws on an aspect of the EMILIA research project, which aimed to gain a better understanding of the impacts of a lifelong learning intervention on the wellbeing of a group of mental health service users. The chapter begins with the introduction of the EMILIA project, the context for the work reported in this chapter. Section two of the chapter interrogates the European Union's rolling definitions/conceptions of lifelong learning with special reference to eight European countries where EMILIA demonstration sites (or pilot implementation centres) were located. Section three highlights lifelong learning provision – the existing lifelong learning intervention as applied to mental health service users – and the paucity of existing provision citing in particular the absence of *targeted* learning that has characterised lifelong learning programmes, courses or training for people with mental illness. Section four presents and discusses the results of the EMILIA project training intervention with a particular focus on qualitative data drawn from interviews with participants at the Middlesex University research site. Finally, the chapter posits the need for funded provision of formal learning and employment opportunities for service users.

Context of study: the EMILIA project

EMILIA is an abbreviation for 'Empowerment of mental illness service users: lifelong learning, integration and action'; it is a framework 6 research and intervention project, funded at €3.4 million over a four and a half year period, from September 2005 to February 2010. The EMILIA project was one of a number of European development programmes funded by the European Union, part of a wider effort to address the problem of exclusion of multiple disadvantaged groups such as the unemployed people with long-term mental health illness. EMILIA was the European Union's largest ever funded research and intervention project on lifelong learning and social inclusion in the mental health area. The project had 16 partners in 13 European countries. A major goal of the project was to explore the use of lifelong learning through *EMILIA intervention activity* or training, as a means of achieving improved social inclusion of people with long-term mental health illness. The EMILIA training programmes were implemented across eight demonstration sites in eight European countries – namely the United Kingdom, France, Norway, Greece, Spain, Poland, Bosnia and Herzegovina and Denmark. The project's ultimate goal was to achieve the integration of European policy in the areas of lifelong learning, social inclusion, employment, and information technology as applied to mental health.

Europe's policy context for lifelong learning

The Lisbon Summit of the European Union heads of states and governments in March 2000 set the policy context for lifelong learning. The Lisbon agenda, as it later become known, set forth an overarching goal of making the European Union region the 'most competitive and dynamic knowledge-driven economy by 2010'. In March 2005, also in Lisbon, the 'original' vision of making the European Union region a most competitive economic block was amplified by the European Council meeting. That meeting brought clarity to the 'original' Lisbon agenda with the addition of a handful of new dimensions, which include social inclusion and community cohesion/citizenship. What is significant to note is that lifelong learning became a linchpin of the economic, social and cultural dimensions of the Lisbon agenda and the European Union Member States were obliged to relate national policy to it. Lifelong learning also became a useful tool for promoting social inclusion of multiple disadvantaged groups such as people with mental illness.

Defining lifelong learning

In its simplest form, lifelong learning can be defined as *learning* from cradle to grave. In this line of definition, lifelong learning sees all learning as a continuum, made up of all learning activity undertaken throughout life, be it formal, informal or non-formal. Also, in this line of definition, lifelong learning will include all learning activity undertaken for personal or professional reasons or both. In conceptualising lifelong learning, the European Union (Com 2001) not only see lifelong learning as a continuum but define it in terms of specific outcomes. According to the European Commission, lifelong learning is 'all learning activity undertaken throughout life, with the aim of improving knowledge, skills and competence, within a personal, civic, social and/or employment-related perspective' (Com 2001). What is clear from the foregoing is that the European Union's definition of lifelong learning consciously highlights priority action areas for Member States to reflect in policy frameworks at the national level. It is not surprising therefore that, at the national level, lifelong learning is defined largely in terms of outcomes – often in terms of economic growth and jobs. For example, in Norway, lifelong learning is conceptualised as a continuum: it is defined as *learning* which provides opportunity for citizens 'to acquire new knowledge and skills throughout life, so that they are able to function well in society and keep up with the constantly changing demands of working life' (Norwegian Ministry of Education and Research 2007). Similarly, in the UK, lifelong learning is twinned with the government's widening participation agenda: both are predicated on economic, cultural and social factors. According to the UK government (DfEE 1998), lifelong learning is 'the continuous development of the skills, knowledge and understanding' that are essential for today's job and personal fulfilment. In other words, in the UK, the economic goal of lifelong learning is as important as the social/citizenship goal. Lifelong learning in Greece, as in the UK, places emphasis both on the economic and social inclusion dimensions, which is broadly in line with the Lisbon agenda. In Greece, therefore, lifelong learning is conceptualised as a 'continuum of the different forms of learning on a life scale,' aimed primarily at enhancing 'the quality of education provision, improving employability, re-skilling the workforce, and [promoting] social inclusion and citizenship' (National Report on Lifelong Learning, Greece 2007). In France, lifelong learning is understood to include 'learning for all at all levels' and every citizen, irrespective of personal circumstances, has a right to lifelong learning. The Danish conception of lifelong learning is a cradle-to-grave approach, from pre-school learning through to higher education and adult education and continuing training; every citizen has a right to attend lifelong learning training and courses, even if the policy framework for lifelong learning tends to be biased towards people in employment. In Spain, lifelong learning is predicated on *learning*, qualification and job-related skills development; it is defined as 'the act of useful learning carried out continuously with the aim of improving qualifications, expanding knowledge and aptitudes (Eve, de Groot and Schmidt 2007). Similarly, in Poland, lifelong learning is defined in terms of specific outcomes: it is a 'process of continued improvement, upgrading or changing the attained educational level, skills and qualifications, and thus adaptation to the changing environment' (Polish Ministry of Economy and Labour 2005). Although not a member of the European Union, Bosnia and Herzegovina is a signatory to the European Union Memorandum for lifelong learning – to that extent it endorses the standard European Union's definition of lifelong learning. Currently, in Bosnia and Herzegovina, lifelong learning is implicitly situated in both adult education and vocational education and training; these are currently not joined up because of an absence of a coherent national strategy for lifelong learning.

It is clear from the foregoing that the conception of lifelong learning at the national level accords broadly with the European Union's lifelong learning agenda as set out in the Lisbon strategy. It is also clear that there are differences between countries in the policy orientation towards lifelong learning: for example, the economic dimension (growth and jobs) and the social/cultural dimension (citizenship and social inclusion) were emphasised as national policy goals, with the economic dimension being on the whole more dominant.

Existing lifelong learning intervention for mental health service users

In terms of the delivery of lifelong learning, there is no standard practice or template across the eight countries. However, across Europe, there are widespread, albeit differing, lifelong learning courses, programmes and training for any interested citizens and residents. In the case of people with mental illness, provision in most cases takes the form of training courses or programmes in formal settings. In the United Kingdom, for example, lifelong learning courses and programmes in many state-funded further education and higher education colleges and universities, local government-funded adult education colleges and centres, and Non-Governmental Organisation [NGO]-run education and training centres reflect broadly the government lifelong learning/widening participation agenda. Lifelong learning courses for mental health service users include basic skills and skill upgrading and development, enabling mental health service users to train to become nurses and teachers or trainers to other service users (Stenfors-Hayes, Griffiths and Ogunleye 2008). There are also opportunities for mental health service users who might want to attend employment and self-employment-related training courses, as part of a strategy to achieve social and professional integration of persons from multiple disadvantaged groups through social enterprise. Eligible mental health service users are also able to attend free or discounted local government-run short courses for pleasure and personal fulfilment, not necessarily leading to qualifications. Across Europe, there are opportunities for mental health service users to attend courses as part of psycho-educational training relevant to their illness, to help them understand or learn about their illness and the strategies needed to recognise and deal with symptoms. Much of this provision relates to basic skills or skill training or job-related skills development, employment training or psycho-education; indeed, in countries such as Greece, for example, a limited number of day education and training centres offered courses in psychoeducation for people with mental illness. Lifelong learning training is also available for service users who wish to acquire life skills, with training programmes or courses in 'social skills' (for example in Poland) and in 'skills for independent living' (for example in the UK).

Gaps in the existing lifelong learning intervention

It is clear that, across Europe, the existing lifelong learning intervention takes the form of a 'one-size-fits-all' approach which does not sufficiently take account of the individual needs of people with mental illness. One reason for a 'one-size-fits-all' approach is that most providers of lifelong learning are mainstream education and training institutions and lifelong learning courses and programmes are generally targeted at mainstream adult learners. It ought to be noted that, across Europe, the funding mechanism for many publicly funded providers of lifelong learning is based on student numbers, retention and progression. These mainstream provider institutions are therefore not able to offer provision that does not lead to qualification for the learner. Other reasons for the paucity of provision include a lack of capacity (insufficient staff expertise in dealing with mental health service users) and a problem of financial resources (more pronounced among providers of lifelong learning in countries such as Greece, Poland and Bosnia and Herzegovina). For service users who are able to work, there are added issues of limited opportunities for employment following a lifelong learning training programme.

The EMILIA intervention

The EMILIA project intervention aimed to address the paucity of *targeted* lifelong learning provision for mental health service users by offering mental health service users formal learning and employment opportunities. The lifelong learning modules which were developed across the project are summarised below:

1. A 'Dual Diagnosis' programme designed for persons living with dual diagnosis to obtain knowledge of how to identify their needs, of the ways to solve problems, to exchange important information with other users and of how to manage their everyday life. One of the main goals of this training is user empowerment.
2. 'Empowering in Recovery' aims to empower mental health service users by increasing their sense of control, give skills to cope with stigma and to improve awareness of positive resources.
3. The aim of the 'Family/Network Support' Training programme is to help students and their support persons (family or close friends) develop skills on how to tackle stress.
4. The aim of the 'Post-Traumatic Stress Support' programme is to enable users and their family members/caretakers to understand the process of traumatisation, and the psychobiological and behavioural consequences of trauma. For users to learn how to migrate these consequences or for their caretakers to support this coping process.
5. 'Powerful Voices' is a mental health service user leadership programme based upon the Consultancy Development Programme. The Course is designed to offer mental health service users the opportunity to take an active part in promoting the mental health service user movement and in bringing the voice of people who use services into every aspect of service development and training. Many people who have completed similar programmes in the UK now occupy leadership positions in local mental health service-user groups. For some people the programme has led to paid work as service-user consultants.
6. The overall purpose of the 'Social Competences' programme is to give the students tools to clarify their job aspirations and the competences they have.

7. The 'Social Network' programme's aim is to equip the students with tools for the construction of a sensitive and effective social network, as well as to belonging to such a network in an active and significant way.

8. 'Building on Personal Strengths'. This 'Strengths Approach' training programme emphasises a process of identifying the strengths, achievements and aspirations of the student. It seeks to enhance the student's capacities to define and meet their needs and aspirations within their own local neighbourhoods and communities both by acting individually and collectively.

9. The aim of the 'Suicide Intervention' programme is to prevent suicide among mental health service users and to stimulate and support self-help of mental health care with users in suicide prevention.

10. The overall aim of the 'User Research Skills' programme is to provide people who use mental health services with an opportunity to develop skills, knowledge and experience in research methods and to gain relevant work experience through their involvement in research project work.

The EMILIA training programmes are available free of charge at www.emiliatraining.net. A toolbox provides instructions for trainers, developed from the experience of the demonstration sites while delivering the training in the EMILIA project. The toolbox provides tips and recommendations for planning and delivering the training, going from who should be offered training, to how to put together a group, advance preparation needed and how to adapt programmes to local needs.

Any of the demonstration sites could select a minimum of three modules from this overall syllabus summarised above. In terms of how this was interpreted and implemented at Middlesex University, four modules were selected. The titles of the core learning modules were 'Building on Strengths and Personal Development Planning', 'Empowering People in Recovery', and 'Powerful Voices: User Leadership and Advocacy'. The additional module was entitled 'User Research Skills'. All teaching was conducted by mental health service users who were leaders in the mental health community – thereby achieving the employment goal of the intervention.

At Middlesex, a certificate of completion, learning support, the option of academic assessment to obtain Middlesex University credits and opportunities and training for paid employment at Middlesex University (teaching and assessing student mental health nurses) were also provided.

Results of the EMILIA intervention at the Middlesex demonstration site

The following discussion uses extracts from the qualitative analysis of data from Middlesex University research site to describe the effects of the EMILIA intervention on participants' wellbeing (names used are anonymised).

> Doing the EMILIA course has given me more confidence in myself and I've realised I can do things even though I struggled.
>
> (Rena)

Having confidence is clearly a valuable resource which enables an individual to mobilise and access other resources. Also within this quote is the mention of persistence despite difficulties, which is a coping strategy often vital to ensure success in life. It is positively linked with confidence, hope and an active optimistic style labelled as 'fighting spirit' (Olason and Rodger 2001). Fighting spirit is linked to adaptive health behaviour and coping with disease (Pettingale, Morris, Greer and Haybittle 1985, Spiegel 2001). Also, in terms of psychological resources, a participant mentioned an increase in dignity and a sense of importance:

> I think that it [EMILIA training] has given me some dignity in my situation [having mental difficulties] and I absolutely hate receiving benefits and I think that it [EMILIA training] has given someone in my position the dignity to feel a bit important anyway.
>
> (Una)

A sense of dignity is part of the human need to achieve and maintain various forms of integrity and it is linked to a sense importance, intrinsic worthiness and self esteem. Deegan (1988) described the mental health recovery as process *'to re-establish a new and valued sense of integrity...'*

Social support has been identified as a key element to recovery (Langeland and Wahl 2009). One participant simply stated that: *'I have made more friends'* (Ben). Another participant stated that EMILIA was useful in terms of: *'... drawing on the support and strengths within the community'* (Dawoh). Yet another participant underlined the value of the social interaction with other service users that contributed towards more positive feelings and their recovery:

> I consider my participation in the EMILIA project to have [...] enabled me to meet and interact with people with similar mental health

issues in a positive and constructive way, that at the time it was happening made me feel better in myself and better able to face up to life in general.

(Norris)

Another key to recovery is motivation: '[Motivation] *developed, it progressed during the training'* (Isabel) and '[EMILIA gave me] *more motivation to pursue and maintain new social contacts'* (Steven). The EMILIA project tried to motivate its participants to pursue and complete the learning programme by connecting the intervention with an individual's personal goals. The following statement is representative of comments expressed in relation to this:

It's all positive stuff. I found that very, very useful in terms of focusing and setting my goals and stuff. It helped to firm up my ideas and goals, I found it very useful.

(Dawoh)

Many participants developed or found goals related to the mental health issues explored in the training, examples of which is provided through the following extracts:

I want to do some voluntary training in order to eventually get paid employment in the mental health field.

(Ben)

I may do something in mental health in the future because I am so passionate about it.

(Isabel)

There were many other statements which revealed insights into the development of goals in other areas. While no claim is made that the project installed all of these goals in the participants, it did help many participants discover and set their own goals. The EMILIA teachers helped participants to understand how the information taught related to real-life issues and the participant's life goals and roles (Parnell 1994).

Connected to the formulation of goals is future orientation. Frankl's (1992) work demonstrated the importance of being 'oriented toward the future, toward a meaning to be fulfilled... in the future' in order be able to successfully adapt and cope in life. The project may have reduced the negative effect of future-orientated uncertainty caused by the experience of mental disorder (McCann and Clark 2004). There were a number of extracts describing future orientation, for example: 'I started to think: "what do I need to do in the next year or so?"' (Ben). Another participant provided a direct reference to increased meaningfulness in their lives that had emerged from their experience of the EMILIA project:

> It [Emilia] has made me feel that what I went through was not in vain if you see what I mean. Because I went through what I went through and I was lucky enough to come out the other end I can help others and that is where I'm from if you see what I mean...
>
> (Alvita)

Helping to achieve a realisation that their experience of mental illness had provided participants with strengths, coping skills and expert knowledge of the health system that can help them in their lives, and also that they could use this experience to help others in their recovery, was one of the core themes of the 'Strengths' module and a goal of the project overall.

Furthermore, taking action to help to develop agency and empowerment can facilitate recovery (Green 2004). There were many comments made in relation to empowerment:

> I have been able to begin to break the social restrictions I grew up with, and take ownership of my life, to build healthier boundaries.
>
> (Steven)

> And also being honest with myself and being able to ask for help when I need it. Because I never used to do that.
>
> (Isabel)

Increased empowerment may have enhanced self-directedness (defined as how responsible, purposeful and resourceful a person is in working to achieve their goals and values). Empowering an individual to take greater responsibility for his or her life unlocks resources and helps create hope for the future (Langeland et al. 2007). Representing the feelings of many, one participant expressed the following:

> Yeah. I am more hopeful for the future.
>
> (Alvita)

Many of the participants gained employment outside of the project, both paid and voluntary, in the 10 months from baseline: four of the participants started to play an active role at a mental health charity, one became an administrator, trustee and legal advisory to a major mental health charity and another successfully helped set up a mental health related social firm. One participant described the benefits that they derived from their new employment:

> It is all about getting back to the helping aspects and I like that. If I do something good in the day it makes me feel good. It makes me feel better.
>
> (Grace)

The analysis revealed that exposure to the EMILIA project also led to the development of existing and new areas of interest for many of its participants, such as interest in the service-user movement, mental health research or the process of recovery. This is likely to have stimulated minds (increasing comprehensibility), enriched lives (increasing meaningfulness) and lead to feelings of personal satisfaction (which can be important in a feeling of confidence).

Many of the extracts in relation to goals, empowerment and areas of interest provide evidence that the EMILIA teachers were able to get participants to see both the specific objectives of learning and the larger meaning as it relates to real-life issues and to participants' actual roles in life. This is what Parnell (1994) describes as essential in effective teaching. It also helps demonstrates that the modules had meaning for those who completed them, that they connected to the participants' needs, problems, preferences, real-world existence, goals and ambitions (Parnell 1994, Boeree 1991).

Increased levels of employment, working towards goals and new areas of interest are all a part of active engagement in life. There is a dynamic positive relationship between active engagement in life and meaningfulness strength (Carstens and Spangenberg 1997, Frankl 1992, Mascaro and Rosen 2005, Yalom 1980).

Increased levels of employment, working towards goals and new areas of interest are also connected to purpose in life. As Mascaro and Rosen (2005) explained, if a person finds increased purpose in life then it is likely that this would strengthen aspects of his or her mental health such as hope, well-being and self confidence.

The analysis of the results revealed extracts relating to eight different examples of this: EMILIA's efforts to develop effective learner teacher relationships; allowing learners to express and validate their concerns and questions; creating a friendly supportive environment; providing constructive feedback; providing opportunities for self reflection; the project's efforts to take into account the needs of users by allowing frequent breaks during the training; the size of the group (approx 10-12 students), which participants generally responded well to; EMILIA group teaching style and its use of variety of methods of delivery of material.

The analysis also highlighted the positive effects of employing mental health service users as trainers which helps confirm Rummel et al. (2005) findings that peer led education for mental health service users is effective. Mental health service-user trainers may have acted as role models, allowing participants to see that others can cope with and be successful despite their mental illness (Ascher-Svanum and Whitesel 1999). Young and Ensing's (1999) literature review found that learning through role models and peers with a similar experience can have an especially large positive effect on recovery. The following extract is representative of participant comments:

> It was good that the teachers were in the same position as us [mental health service users] as well. That was very good. I think that that helped [us] to open up. I think that if the teachers hadn't experienced mental ill health, I would have probably opened up but perhaps some other people may not have done. That was a very good [aspect to the training]. It gave me more of a push to achieve as well.

> (Alvita)

Most participants stuck with the project despite the challenges and problems which they faced. Research suggests that successful coping can lead to the development of further adaptive coping resources (Aldwin 2000). There is evidence from the qualitative analysis that EMILIA had a positive effect on mental health recovery:

> EMILIA had an [positive] impact. It came at a time when I was transitioning and it helped with the transition. The EMILIA strengths training help[ed] with my transitioning and focus on positive goals drawing on community supports.

> (Dawoh)

> I consider my participation in the EMILIA project to have gone well... that at the time it was happening, it made me feel better in myself and better able to face up to life in general.

> (Norris)

Sharing in the group activities, learning things about myself that I didn't know. I thought I had a lot of things down in my mind about how I was and how I came to be here but I didn't really. And learning different things and challenging myself. Things that I never thought I would do. It is changing and it is a positive change.

(Isabel)

The recovery associated extracts support the findings of Borg and Kristiansen (2008) that employment, learning, and social interaction are all important in generating a sense of hope, meaning, wellbeing and self-esteem. The extracts also reflect the core recovery processes identified by Green (2004): development, learning, healing and adaption. Charmaz (1991) describes recovery as involving the development of an understanding of abilities and limitations (comprehensibility factor), making adaptations and day-to-day life management decisions (manageability factor) and setting long term goals that take into account the reality faced in terms of strengths and capabilities (meaningfulness factor).

The results of this study link recovery, social inclusion and lifelong learning; these support the findings of Hammond (2004) that learning can have positive impact upon factors that include self-esteem, self-efficacy, a sense of purpose and hope, competences, and social integration. The results also support the findings of Feinstein and Hammond (2004) that participation in formal learning is an important element in positive cycles of personal and social development and progression.

Concluding remarks

Promoting the social inclusion of disadvantaged groups such as people with mental illness remains a commitment at the European level. The funding of a number of European development projects – including EMILIA – further underpins this commitment. Despite national differences in the policy orientation towards lifelong learning, there is a broad alignment to the European Union's conception of lifelong learning as set out in the Lisbon strategy. The progress that has been made in terms of the alignment of lifelong learning policy at national level has not translated into practical reality for mental health service users (Stenfors-Hayes, Griffiths and Ogunleye 2008). The fact is that, across Europe, existing provision takes the form of 'one-size-fits-all', an approach that does not sufficiently take account of the particular needs and desires of service users.

The absence of *targeted* lifelong learning interventions for service users has created a gap which the EMILIA intervention aimed to bridge by offering mental health service users formal learning and employment opportunities. The analysis of the EMILIA intervention indicates support for the funding and delivery of programmes such as EMILIA which can be considered part of the responsibility of society to empower mental health service users. Projects such as EMILIA offer the opportunity to participate in a normalising activity and thus help to reduce the problem of social marginalisation experienced by so many people with severe and enduring mental health disorders. The findings provide evidence for continued and embedded use of the modules designed for the EMILIA project and for extending EMILIA's underlying principles and practical application to further groups of mental health service users. Project such as EMILIA could be implemented across and beyond Europe.

An EMILIA-style opportunity could be an integrated part of mental health services. Mental health service users could be offered a choice of different learning modules, and on completion of these they could be offered help in finding a job and supported in the competitive market place. Providing embedded, EMILIA-style opportunities requires among others, adequate funding, cooperation between health services, education providers and integrated and progressive systems that are sensitive to the individual, their needs and their right to be socially included.

Acknowledgements

This study is funded by the European Union under its 6th Framework Programme. EMILIA (Empowerment of Mental Illness Service Users: Life Long Learning, Integration and Action), CIT 3-CT-2005-513435.

References

Aldwin, C. M. (2000). *Stress, Coping and Development: An Integrative Perspective* (New York: Guilford Press).

Ascher-Svanum, H. and Whitesel, J. (1999). 'A Randomized Controlled Study of Two Styles of Group Patient Education about Schizophrenia', *Psychiatric Services*, L, 926–30.

Boere, C. G. (1991). 'Teaching for Meaning', *Journal of Professional Studies*, 15, http://webspace.ship.edu/cgboer/meaning.html, date accessed 14 June 2011.

Borg, M. and Kristiansen, K. (2008). 'Working on the Edge: The Meaning of Work for People Recovering from Severe Mental Distress in Norway', *Disability & Society*, XXIII, (5), 511–23.

Carstens, J. A. and Spangenberg, J. J. (1997). 'Major Depression: A Breakdown in Sense of Coherence?' *Psychological Reports*, LXXX, 1211–20.

Charmaz, K. (1991). *Good Days; Bad Days: The Self in Chronic Illness* (New Jersey: Rutgers University Press).

Deegan, P. E. (1988). 'Recovery: The Lived Experience of Rehabilitation', *Psychosocial Rehabilitation Journal*, XI, 11–19.

DfEE (1998). 'The Learning Age: A Renaissance for a New Britain' (London: Department for Education and Employment).

EU COM (2001). 'Communication for the Commission, Making a European Area of Lifelong Learning a Reality' (Luxembourg: European Commission, November).

Eve, J., de Groot, M. and Schmidt, A. M. (2007). 'Supporting Lifelong Learning in Public Libraries across Europe', *Library Review*, LVI, 5, 393–406. www. emeraldinsight.com/Insight/ViewContentServlet?Filename=Published/ EmeraldFullTextArticle/Articles/0350560505.html, date accessed 8 March 2009.

Feinstein, L. and Hammond, C. (2004). 'The Contribution of Adult Learning to Health and Social Capital', *Oxford Review of Education*, XXX, 199–221.

Frankl, V. E. (1992). *Man's Search for Meaning*, 3rd edn (London: Hodder & Stoughton).

Greece Ministry of Education (2007). National Report on the Implementation of the Education and Training 2010 Work Programme. http://ec.europa.eu/ education/policies/2010/natreport07/el_en.pdf, accessed 19 February 2009.

Green, C. A. (2004). 'Fostering Recovery from Life-Transforming Mental Health Disorders: A Synthesis and Model', *Social Theory and Health*, II, 293–314.

Hammond, C. (2004). 'Impacts of Lifelong Learning upon Emotional Resilience, Psychological and Mental Health: Fieldwork Evidence', *Oxford Review of Education*, XXX, 551–68.

Langeland, E. and Wahl, A. (2009). 'The Impact of Social Support on Mental Health Service Users' Sense of Coherence: A Longitudinal Panel Survey', *International Journal of Nursing Studies*, XLVI, 6, 830–7.

Langeland, E., Wahl, A. K., Kristoffersen, K, Nortvedt, M. and Hanestad, B. R. (2007). 'Sense of Coherence Predicts Change in Life Satisfaction among Home-Living Residents in the Community with Mental Health Problems: A 1-Year Follow-up Study', *Quality of Life Research*, XVI, 6, 939–46.

Mascaro, N. and Rosen, D. H. (2005). 'Existential Meaning's Role in the Enhancement of Hope and Prevention of Depressive Symptoms', *Journal of Personality*, LXXIII, 985–1013.

McCann, T. V. and Clark, E. (2004). 'Embodiment of Severe and Enduring Mental Illness: Finding Meaning in Schizophrenia', *Issues in Mental Health Nursing*, XXIV, 783–98.

Norwegian Ministry of Education (2007). National Report on the Implementation of the Education and Training 2010 Work Programme Norway, http:// ec.europa.eu/education/policies/2010/natreport07/no_en.pdf, date accessed 19 February 2009.

Olason, D. T. and Roger, D., (2001). 'Optimism, Pessimism and "Fighting Spirit": A New Approach to Assessing Expectancy and Adaptation', *Personality and Individual Differences*, XXXI, 5, 755–68.

Parnell, D. (1994). *LogoLearning: Searching for Meaning in Education* (Waco, Texas: Cord Communications).

Pettingale, K. W., Morris, T., Greer, S. and Haybittle, J. L. (1985). 'Mental Attitudes to Cancer: An Additional Prognostic Factor', *Lancet*, I, 750.

Polish Ministry of Economy and Labour (2005). *Employment in Poland 2005*, Department of Economic Analyses and Forecasts, Ministry of Economy and Labour, M. Bukowski (ed). ISBN 83-60302-15-4.

Rummel, C. B., Hansen, W. P., Helbig, A., Pitschel-Walz, G. and Kissling, W. (2005). 'Peer-to-Peer Psychoeducation in Schizophrenia: A New Approach', *The Journal of Clinical Psychiatry*, LXVI, 1580–5.

Spiegel, D. (2001). 'Mind Matters: Coping and Cancer Progression', *Journal of Psychosomatic Research*, L, 5, 287–90.

Stenfors-Hayes, T., Griffiths, C. and Ogunleye, L (2008). 'Lifelong Learning for all? Policies, Barriers and Practical Reality for a Socially Excluded Group', *International Journal of Lifelong Education*, XXVII, 6, 625–40.

Yalom, I. D. (1980). *Existential Psychotherapy* (New York: Basic Books).

Young, S. L. and Ensing, D. S. (1999). 'Exploring Recovery from the Perspective of People with Psychiatric Disabilities', *Psychiatric Rehabilitation Journal*, XXII, 3, 19–32.

13
Stakeholders' Lifelong Learning and Organisational Change Experiences in the Context of the EMILIA Project

Marja Kaunonen and Shulamit Ramon

This chapter will focus on presenting the research evidence pertaining to the centrality of lifelong learning in organisations involved in mental health service provision and education. Use will be made of an extensive international literature review on the topic, of data drawn from the EMILIA project on this theme, and of our wider personal-professional experience of working in mental health and educational settings. EMILIA's research utilised the five-stage process anchored in the European Union's lifelong learning policy (EU 2001). The first stage identifies *partnership working across the learning spectrum*, according to which all actors inside and outside the formal systems must collaborate in the development of learning organisations for strategies to work. Stage 2 is concerned with *insight into demand for learning*, which EMILIA operationalised by carrying out systematic lifelong learning needs assessments of the mental health service users. Stage 3, *Analysis, generation and development of adequate financial and learning resources for the task*, is concerned with the institutional resourcing of the lifelong learning assessed as needed in the previous stage. Stage 4 is entitled *Facilitating user access to learning and work opportunities*. This stage proceeds to match learning opportunities to learners' needs and to facilitate access to the learning opportunities the users themselves have selected locally. Finally, stage 5, *Striving for excellence through service improvement*, ensures that a comprehensive integrated approach to lifelong learning (and social inclusion) is in place in the institutions concerned. European lifelong learning policy (EU 2011) assumes that the point of departure is for any service organisation focused upon to become a learning organisation, due to the inter-relationships between organisations, people who

189

use their services, and those who work for/in them. Using as a case study data drawn from the eight demonstration sites in the EMILIA project (Empowerment of Mental Service Users: Lifelong Learning, Integration and Action, EU Contract Number 513435), we will discuss whether the eight demonstration sites have become learning organisations, the extent of moving in this direction, the obstacles and opportunities met in this process and the degree to which they meet the different facets of lifelong learning. We will then analyse how the organisational experience was connected to the extent of the lifelong learning that took place in the life of individual members of the project. Finally we will look at whether power has shifted from the organisation towards mental health service users as reflected in their new activities and views, applying Foucault's (1972 and 1977) conceptualisation of positive power.

Introduction

The EMILIA project, funded by the EU under its Framework 6 between 2005–2010, recruited adults (age 18 and above), diagnosed as having severe and enduring mental illness (schizophrenia and bipolar disorder), in contact with mental health services for at least three years and who were not in paid employment. They were offered a series of training modules, social activities with other service users, and attempts were made to offer them employment opportunities within the demonstration sites and to connect them to potential employers outside the sites in which the project operated (Athens, Barcelona, Bodø, London, Paris, Tuzla, Warsaw and Zealand).

An extensive quantitative and qualitative evaluation took place at baseline, 10 months and 20 months points in time, of mental health service users' sociodemographic state, their take up of the training and of unpaid and paid employment, their own evaluation of the impact of participation in the project in relation to employment, social interaction, training activities, opportunities and obstacles, and goals for the near future.

The focus of the EMILIA project on enhancing social inclusion and recovery for people with long term mental illness called for a process of adaptation in the demonstration sites, given that meeting these objectives required an organisational structure and atmosphere that not only welcomed service users but also was ready to offer them opportunities far beyond those usually on offer in clinical practice in preparing them for a more independent life, employment, and enhancing their social network as means of empowerment (Ramon et al. 2011, Ramon 2011).

With this need in mind, the research team constructed the organisational case study in parallel to the service-user case study, to enable us to follow this process and to collect data representing its development. The data collection measures included

- Recorded observations of key project group meetings at baseline, after the first 10 months and after 20 months.
- Recorded focus groups at the same points in time.
- Organisational documentary data, such as strategy.

The rationale for selecting these measures has been in part the wish to use existing opportunities where organisational change will be demonstrated, such as in the meetings of the sites' steering groups and the documentary data. The focus group method was added as an opportunity for reflection for the steering group, and was preferred to individual interviews as most of the project activities were conducted in groups (Kitzinger 1994, Morgan 1996). The focus groups were specifically convened to provide feedback on the project, whereas the observations relate to meetings due to take place in any case.

Throughout the project, the eight demonstration sites varied considerably in culture, economic position, the structure of mental health services, in readiness and ability to offer genuine social inclusion and recovery opportunities to people with severe mental illness experience. Only the last two variables will be looked at in this text. Each of the sites had to make the effort to find meaningful training, activities and employment opportunities for the recruited service users who met the project's inclusion criteria, mentioned above.

Seven of the sites were providing mental health services, while one site was a university faculty (London); two of the clinical sites were also research centres (Zealand in Denmark and Warsaw in Poland). Of the seven sites, five had a hospital as the core of their service, and three had community services such as day centre and group homes (Athens, Greece), a users group (Tuzla, Bosnia), and an out-patient clinic (Zealand). It is interesting to note that these differences did, and did not, impact on the ability of a site to provide these opportunities. The more advanced sites in terms of offering the more empowering training and work opportunity were the university site, a hospital based site, and the service-cum-research centre. Moreover, although based in a fairly traditionally medicalised organisation, the hospital site was also the more innovative site in terms of mainstreaming gender and ethnicity (Ramon et al. 2010).

It would therefore seem that what enables sites to change in the direction required by the aims of the project has less to do with its formal structure and more with other factors, hopefully revealed in the data collected from observations and focus groups. Our interest in organisational change related also to the focus on lifelong learning (LLL) as the EU preferred framework for the implementation of the project, and consequently on each site as a learning organisation (LO). It is with these two concepts in mind that we have approached our analysis of organisational change.

This text will focus on organisational change as a necessary but insufficient condition for the implementation of social inclusion and recovery in practice. Organisational change will be treated as a process variable, namely as a component needed for the success of any fundamental change in human services that requires a multi-level shift in values, knowledge and skills.

It is assumed here that such a process is necessary to facilitate the unlearning and re-learning which social inclusion and recovery implementation entails for both individual practitioners as key stakeholders and the organisation in which they work.

The challenge encountered in implementing social inclusion and recovery highlights that a number of areas would require change in attitudes, knowledge and skills as highlighted by a number of researchers and activists in this field (Davidson 2003, Ramon 2005, Rapp and Goscha 2006, Deegan and Drake 2006).

The individualised nature of the process of recovery requires a high degree of flexibility and a system evolving around meeting individualised needs and wishes, and presents a challenge for services built to meet the needs of sub-groups, rather than individualised care.

Furthermore, taking into account the multiplicity of the stakeholders involved (users, carers, professionals, managers, commissioners, politicians, the general public) makes the demand on the organisation even more complex than it would have been otherwise.

The introduction of social inclusion and recovery is likely to be perceived as a threat to a large number of mental health professionals who continue to believe in the traditional perspective of mental illness. Moreover, it is likely to be seen as a threat also to the many service users who have internalised the self identity of the chronically sick person incapable of living well with the illness and of developing a life beyond the illness (Henderson 2011).

Approaches to organisational change

There are a number of approaches to organisational change, recognised as a central component to achieving success in the current highly changeable, uncertain and competitive organisational climate. Two of them are presented here because of their potential contribution to a more in-depth understanding of organisational change within socially inclusive, recovery-oriented practice.

• Focus on the Learning Organisation as the major vehicle for change as highlighted by Senge (1990) and by Birleson, Brann and Smith (2001).
• Complexity Theory approach to the diffusion of innovation (McLaughlin and Paton 2008).

The first approach tends to treat the introduction of change as an exercise in good management. Organisations need to become good learning organisations (Argyris and Schon 1978, 1996, Gould and Baldwin 2004) if they are to survive and succeed in rapidly changing societies.

More specifically, the LO has to develop systemic thinking, personal mastery, challenge ingrained mental models, build a shared vision, and team learning through dialogue, if it is to build a culture of innovation (Senge et al. 1994). Leaders need to be designers, stewards (serving the organisation and its membership) and teachers (Senge 1990).

To build a learning organisation, three types of leadership, spread over the whole organisation, are essential (Senge 1996, Birleson, Brann and Smith 2001):

1. Local line leaders, who undertake meaningful organisational experiments to test the effectiveness of new learning capabilities.
2. Executive leaders who support line-leaders, develop learning infrastructures and lead by example.
3. Internal networkers, or community builders whose role is to spot those more ready for change, help in organisational experiments, and aid the diffusion of new learning.

The importance of maintaining continuous change, and the difficulties this entails have been highlighted by Handy (1989). Coming from the

194 Lifelong Learning and Organisational Change

mental health field, Birleson, Brann and Smith (2001) perceived the key characteristics of the learning organisation to include, in addition to leadership, organisational and work design, experimentation, information processing and communication.

The approach is attractive in its focus on the ideal collective learning organisation focused on both innovation and the future, and has applications for business organisations as well as human services organisations (Gould and Baldwin 2004), though the application to each of them should not be treated as synonymous given the difference in focus of the LO's core vision and activity. However, the concept as outlined by Senge (1990) does not take into account the social relations that exist in such an organisation (Gheradi 1999). It also ignores the short-term thinking prevalent in most business oriented organisations which focus on improving their financial profits, and the ensuing lack of attention to collective reflection and learning.

Likewise, the lack of commitment to a specific change by the majority of members of the organisation, and the emotional ramifications change brings about are treated as issues which do not deserve much attention. The political dimension is disliked and a fear of conflict as a mode of relationships within organisations seems to prevail (Sennett 1998).

The diffusion of the innovatory elements of social inclusion and recovery principles and ways of working is at the heart of the organisational change required in this case. Hence there is a need to look at approaches to the diffusion of innovation. We shall focus on the complexity approach to the diffusion of innovation (McLaughlin and Paton 2008) as it is more comprehensive than other related models, and does not approach the diffusion as a linear process. This approach to the diffusion of innovation stresses the importance of the relative advantage of the proposed change, its compatibility with the values an organisation or an individual holds, relevant past experiences, its complexity, trialability and observability which make the difference as to whether one is/is not ready to adopt a change (McLaughlin and Paton 2008).

The realisation that organisational change is almost inevitably disruptive, even when desired, has been focused upon by theorists of the complexity approach such as Ferlie et al. (2005). The disruption is to interpersonal relations, group boundaries, professional roles and identities. Thus, paying attention to role transition becomes an important part of the process (Bridges 2002), as does the emotional aspect of organisational change. Often, the latter is not treated as an integral part of the process of change (Hargreaves 1998), leading Fineman (2005) to state that usually organisations treat change as 'emotionally anorexic'. Research on organisational change in health settings highlights the high likelihood of it evolving not as predicted, often with chaotic stages which do not necessarily imply lack of effectiveness (Greenhalgh, Robert and Bate 2005).

Both social inclusion and recovery call for a radical departure from the previous mould of mental health services and the ethos of our professional roles, as they require a fundamental shift in the way professionals view service users. It also implies a redistribution of the power relations between users and professionals, in the way working together, and in the way mental illness is perceived. Therefore the complexity theory approach to innovation offers a realistic framework to the diffusion of innovation to recovery implementation than the more idealistic LO perspective.

Organisational change as reflected in the focus groups, documentation and observations

Local research workers were trained to carry out focus groups during a research training week in 2006. The list of themes to be covered in each focus group at baseline, 10 and 20 months periods was prepared by the central researchers in consultation with the local research workers, as was the template for data coding. Thematic analysis (Braun and Clarke, 2006) was applied to this primarily qualitative data.

For most of the time participation in the focus groups was unproblematic; from time to time some participants were unclear about some of the themes and questions. It is unclear whether this reflects the fact that new people joined the focus groups at both 10 and 20 months points, who were usually unaware of the themes already discussed in previous focus groups.

Baseline issues

The key questions asked at baseline inquired about the meaning attached to LLL, how LLL should manifest itself within the LO and by individuals within the LO, opportunities and obstacles within and outside of the LO for the application of LLL, and where would the organisation wish to be in two years time. At baseline, focus groups consisted of members of the steering group of each site, who were usually the key professionals involved in the project and their team members. Most groups had usually up to 10 members.

At that point in time only one site had a service user as a member (London, the university site). This site was also the only one to engage service users in training, and had at the time the possibility of paying for their involvement from the learning and teaching centre they were part of.

Steering group members of all sites were excited by the prospect that the project was offering, but also apprehensive about the enormity of the task ahead. Initial ideas of what each site may provide were mentioned; members of the steering groups were hazy as to what LLL and LO meant, and how these would be facilitated either organisationally or individually. Each site was previously engaged in some attempts at social inclusion, but recovery and empowerment were largely new concepts.

By ten months, the following changes have taken place

A much wider range of participants were present in the focus groups, including mental health professionals (nurses, psychologists and psychiatrists, very few social workers or occupational therapists); heads of services; service users (in two sites for the first time), researchers, university representatives (not only in the university demonstration site), and representatives of external organisations (adult education, minority adult education, job counsellors, carers organisation).

The prominence of user involvement and its highly positive effect on nearly all of the participants in the focus groups has become the new organising focus of LLL within the project, and has led to identifying the creation of opportunities for user involvement at all levels, engaging relevant external organisations (and the media in some sites) to become the new mode of facilitating LLL.

The contribution of the EMILIA project to LLL was perceived mostly as positive, but at times it was felt that it was less effective in preparing people to go back to work. It was helpful to realise through face to face meetings with people from other EMILIA sites that the similarities among sites were greater than the differences. It also was good to realise that staff-user relationships have changed positively, for example through having users as co-researchers and co-trainers.

New internal opportunities have been utilised, such as further development of the annual user conferences, intention to employ users in mental health services (Barcelona, Bodø, Zealand), more teaching opportunities, and training as co-trainers, accreditation of courses.

To these were added some new external opportunities such as the positive involvement of external organisations, such as job counsellors (Paris), school for health services training (Barcelona) and youth centres for social inclusion purposes and working with families (Paris, Barcelona).

Some continuities were commented upon, such as the continuation of the steps to ensure more, and more systematic opportunities for user involvement; use of reflection of the self in a problematic situation of being unwell to that of a service user; providing individual coaching by job counsellors to the satisfaction of most – but not all – service users.

This came together with the continuation of the resistance to change by some staff members, who expressed it as doubts about the users' ability to be involved and to move towards recovery, and fear of their 'fragility' (psychologists in Barcelona and in Paris). Continued old obstacles included stigma both inside the health system and outside it, slow reform process, lack of co-ordination, a fragmented system lacking a good information component, limited funding options, and lack of integration of rehabilitation-focused services, the very long process of change and the inevitable collective and at times individual setbacks.

New internal obstacles had cropped up too, such as the difficulties to offer payment for one-off contribution to teaching by service users; time and staff limitations (Barcelona, Bodø, Paris), prolonged impact of service restructuring (Zealand).

These were combined with new external obstacles, such as no renewed funding for transportation for service users (Tuzla), realising that other parts of the health system accept users as expert patients but not its mental health component due to fears of risk (Barcelona); resistance outside of the faculty (London), reduced opening hours of mental health services.

The major issues at the 20-month point

The focus groups data shows primarily a consolidation of the changes occurring during the first 10 months period. This is reflected in the increased number of service users involved, and a further increase in the number of new people from both inside and outside of the organisation joining in. For a few, but not all sites, there is a change in the meaning of LifeLong Learning in the sense given to EMILIA's activities by both users and providers. Users begin to see their participation in a programme such as EMILIA as a right; both staff and users see the benefits of the training that was offered, and in a number of sites they are attempting to ensure that the training continues for both groups. Pertaining to mode of facilitation of LLL, more users have become involved as trainers or service providers in the sites and in related services, albeit in small numbers (experts by experience in Barcelona, user trainer on a ward in Bodø, Personal Medicine Coaches in Zealand, service-user trainers in London), as well as increased self-confidence by users working in the sites (London), providing training to additional groups such as carers and nurses (Warsaw).

New internal opportunities included users asking for new programmes, establishing a social co-operative (Athens), establishing new settings for the continuation of the training, expansion of opportunities pertaining to involvement in teaching (London), being offered participation in training and conferences as a reward (London, Bodø), more employment opportunities within the site (Paris) and outside it (Zealand, new emergency room project), submission for funding for three new projects prepared by service users (Tuzla).

New external opportunities entailed a variety of options from establishing a close link to other organisations (the Bonanova School in Barcelona, the Birmingham Mental Health Development Centre with Middlesex University and links with the regional carer organisation in Paris), to expanding the range of LLL activities (for example, place and train scheme in Paris) and plans to do so (create a users' umbrella organisation in Tuzla, learning from other experts by experience in Barcelona).

New external obstacles included some new national policies (for example, changes in benefit policy in England); a national system which is not geared to enable independent living for resettled patients (Athens); no resources for LLL, difficulties in finding jobs for users to suit their wishes and skills (Paris).

Old obstacles re-emerging included ignorance, lack of readiness by professionals to collaborate with users (Tuzla), slow pace of mental health reforms, mental illness itself, not enough resources (Bodø and Warsaw), the fragmentation of the system (Paris), the difficulty to innovate within a system which is old and resistant to change (Zealand), a system lacking in transparency, time and staff (Warsaw), the difficulty professionals have in seeing users as trainers (Athens, Barcelona) and in not seeing carers as a resource, lack of flexibility of professionals and the organisation (Bodø).

Ways to resolve obstacles entail addressing lack of time either by extra pay and/or moving activities to other organisations (Barcelona); negotiations (Paris), looking for policies which offer new options (Paris, re benefits). However, it is clear that for a number of obstacles no solutions are likely to emerge in the near future.

The eight demonstration sites achieved a number of their longer term aspirations. These included opening a new co-operative (Athens), completing a training module, beginning to train users to become trainers, and introducing lifelong learning training to the day hospital (Barcelona), preparing and introducing the new figure of expert by experience (Barcelona), users working more days than before (Paris) and EMILIA having a positive image among users and professionals (Paris), the organisation receiving two small grants and submitting two proposals for new projects (Tuzla), and a manual on how to foster recovery being published in the site language (Warsaw).

Development after the EMILIA project

As sites were approaching the end of the project, the near future became a looming issue. A large number of suggestions were made focused on continuing to meet EMILIA's objectives. These included accepting users as employees in the sites, providing further targeted training to both staff and users, establishing structural measures to achieve objectives (London), creating wider networks which offer more pressure power, informing the public and politicians, and supporting further the development of LLL for both users and staff (for example, in the rural areas of Poland, not only in the cities) or applying for new funding (London).

The process of intervention by EMILIA providers

On the whole, this was perceived to be positive by the majority of service users, carers and the range of providers. They liked the interactive nature of the training and being a model of user involvement. The few critical comments concerned specific issues, such as the need to fill in the content of the training modules sent from the co-ordinators of training, not everything being easy to understand for the users, and not all elements being equally innovative.

Usefulness of the EMILIA training programme for other deprived groups

Most sites expressed a firm belief that the training programme would be useful to other deprived groups, across the range of health disabilities (e.g people with addictions (including smoking), with physical and learning difficulties), extended to young offenders, war veterans and older people.

The organisational change was also explored through the documentation of each organisation. The comparison of the documentation at baseline and at the end of the follow up period highlights that the follow up period was limited and changes in the organisations did not reach the documentation layer. This is in line with previous organisational research results indicating that organisational change is a lengthy process and takes more than the EMILIA study's follow-up time of 20 months. Staff meeting observations provided a snapshot of the organisation at the EMILIA study's follow-up points as experienced by its employees, utilised to evaluate the attitudes of the organisation and its professional staff towards employing service users. These attitudes changed between the baseline and the 10 month evaluation point in all participating sites. At the 20 month point, user involvement was taken almost for granted as a positive attribute in nearly all sites. However, while a number of sites had made considerable progress in relation to this aspect, other sites had not. The differences seemed to lie in staff attitudes and cultural context attitudes. On the whole, the EMILIA sites did very well in terms of increased and more varied user involvement, and were good at holding at bay negative attitudes.

Concluding comments

All of the demonstration sites introduced innovations as part of their participation in the EMILIA project. In this sense, the principles of LLL and LO were useful in enabling the implementation of social inclusion and recovery principles in those practice areas of the sites in which EMILIA members were engaged, as highlighted in the evidence illustrated in the focus groups data. At this stage, we lack evidence as to whether these changes will be sustained or not.

Some sites innovated more than others both quantitatively and qualitatively, the degree of which being partly related to the opportunities and obstacles a specific site was confronted with. The extent and depth of obstacles confronted by the users group in Bosnia was particularly harsh in comparison with other sites, while they made a number of valiant attempts that did not seem to alter the situation. Likewise, some of the structural obstacles met by the Greek site were extremely difficult to change. Bearing these constraints in mind while attempting to analyse the focus groups data from the perspective of organisational change, it would appear that several factors facilitated the move towards LLL, and for the organisation to become an LO within the context of the EMILIA project. These factors included transformational leadership of professionals, service users and managers (Ashcraft and Anthony 2005, Benis 2009), readiness to take calculated risks so vital in positive mental health work (Ramon 2005), and working within a society/community/generalised climate in which socio-cultural change was taking place and largely welcomed.

The LLL aspects within the two sets of data discussed in this chapter indicate that both EMILIA users and staff continued their LLL journey at the 20 month point too, looking for new opportunities, focusing on finding a job, taking more personal responsibility, and an active minority ready to do their best to continue with EMILIA activities after the project was over. The project was perceived to have been a very positive experience, with considerable positive impact, reflected in the findings that even after 20 months there was still a motivation for further training. We wonder if indeed training had continued for longer, would there have been even more positive results?

As already mentioned above in the introduction, the more innovative sites were not of the same/similar mould, but rather different in their formal organisational structures. This finding illustrates well the value of the factors just outlined above in terms of their validity to lead to positive change despite the large number of obstacles each site had to overcome or at least neutralise in order to be able to innovate. It also implies that these are factors worth cultivating in mental health organisations that wish to lead to such change, to foster LLL for service users and staff, and to maintain the organisation as a learning organisation.

Methodologically, the organisational case study has been vindicated as part of a learning discourse tool (Boje, 1994), as it provided the LO with feedback three times within the lifetime of the project that it could use to reflect upon and improve its course of action.

References

Argyris, C. and Schon, D. (1978). *Organisational Learning: A Theory of Action Perspective* (Reading, Mass: Addison Wesley).

Argyris, C. and D. Schon (1996). *Organizational Learning II: Theory, Method, and Practice* (Reading, Mass: Addison-Wesley).

Ashcraft, L., and Anthony, W. (2005). 'A Story of Transformation: An Agency Fully Embraces Recovery', *Behavioural Health Care Tomorrow*, XIV, 12–22.

Birleson, P., Brann, P. and Smith, A. (2001). 'Using Program Theory to Develop Key Performance Indicators for Child and Adolescent Mental Health Services', *Australian Health Review* XXIV(1), 10–21.

Benis, W. (2009). *On Becoming a Leader* (New York: Basic Books).

Boje, D. M. (1994). 'Organisational Storytelling: The Struggles of Pre-Modern, Modern, and Postmodern Organisational Learning Discourses', *Management Learning*, XXV (3), 433–61.

Braun, V. and Clarke, V. (2006). 'Using Thematic Analysis in Psychology', *Qualitative Research in Psychology*, III, 77–101.

Bridges, W. (2002). *Managing Transitions: Making the Most of Change* (New York: Perseus Press).

Davidson, L. (2003). *Living Outside Mental Illness: Qualitative Studies of Recovery in Schizophrenia* (New York: New York University Press).

Deegan, P. E. and Drake, R. E. (2006). 'Shared Decision Making and Medication Management in the Rehabilitation Process', *Psychiatric Services*, LVII, 1636–9.

EU (2001). *Communication for the Commission, Making a European Area of Lifelong Learning a Reality* (Luxembourg: European Commission).

EU (2011). *The Lifelong Learning Programme*, www. ec.europa.eu/llp, date accessed: 13 February 2011.

Ferlie, E., Lynn Jr, L. E. and Pollitt, C. (2005). *The Oxford Handbook of Public Management* (New York: Oxford University Press).

Fineman, S. (2005). 'Appreciating Emotions at Work: Paradigm Tensions', *International Journal of Work Organisation and Emotion*, I, 1, 4–19.

Foucault, M. (1972). *The Archaeology of Knowledge* (London: Tavistock).

Foucault, M. (1977). *Discipline and Punishment: The Birth of the Prison* (Harmondsworth: Penguin).

Gheradi, S. (1999). 'Learning as Problem-Driven or Learning in the Face of Mystery', *Organisational Studies*, XX, 1, 101–24.

Gould, N. and Baldwin, M. (ed.) (2004). *Social Work, Critical Reflection and the Learning Organisation* (Aldershot: Ashgate Publishing).

Greenhalgh, T., Robert, G. and Bate, S. P. (2005). *Diffusion of Innovation in Health Services* (Oxford: Blackwells).

Handy, C. (1989). *The Age of Unreason* (London: Arrow Business Books).

Hargreaves, A. (1998). 'The Emotions of teaching and Educational Change' in A. Hargreaves (ed.). *International Handbook of Educational Change* (London: Khnver Academic Publisher), 558–75.

Henderson, A. R. (2011). 'A Substantive Theory of Recovery from the Effects of Severe Persistent Mental Illness', *International Journal of Social Psychiatry*, 57, 2, 564–73.

Kitzinger, J. (1994). 'The Methodology of Focus Groups: The Importance of Interaction between Research Partners', *Sociology of Health and Illness*, XVI, 103–21.

McLaughlin, S. and Paton, R. A. (2008). 'Identifying Barriers that Impact Knowledge Creation and Transfer within Complex Organisation', *Journal of Knowledge Management* XII, 2, 107–23.

Morgan, D. L. (1996). 'Focus Groups', *Annual Review of Sociology*, XXII, 129–52.

Ramon, S. (2005). 'From Risk Taking to Risk Avoidance in Multidisciplinary Mental Health', in J. Tew (ed.). *Social Perspectives in Mental Health* (London: Jessica Kingsley), 184–99.

Ramon, S., Ryan, P. and Urek, M. (2010). 'Attempting to Mainstream Ethnicity in a Multi-Country EU Mental Health and Social Inclusion Project: Lessons for Social Work', *European Journal of Social Work*, XIII, 2, 163–82.

Ramon, S., Griffiths, C., Nieminen, I., Pederson, M. L. and Dawson, I. (2011), 'Towards Social Inclusion through Lifelong Learning in Mental Health: Analysis of Change in the Lives of the EMILIA Project Service Users', *International Journal of Social Psychiatry*, 57, 3, 211–23.

Ramon, S. (2011). 'Organisational Change in the Context of Recovery-Oriented Services', *Journal of Mental Health Workforce Training, Education and Practice* VI, 1, 38–46.

Rapp, C. A. and Goscka, R. J. (2006). *The Strengths Model: Case Management for People with Psychiatric Disabilities*, 2nd edn (Oxford: Oxford University Press).

Sennett, R. (1998). *The Corrosion of Character: The Personal Consequences in the New Capitalism* (New York: Norton).

Senge, P. (1990). *The Fifth Discipline: The Art and Practice of Learning Organisations* (New York: Doubleday).

Senge, P., Kleiner, A., Roberts, C., Ross, R., Roth, G. and Smith, B. (1994). *The Fifth Discipline: Strategies and Tools for Building a Learning Organisation* (New York: Doubleday).

Senge, P. (1996). 'Leading Learning Organisations: The Bold, the Powerful and the Invisible', in R. Goldsmith and G. Hesselbein (eds). *The Leader of the Future* (San Francisco: Jossey Bass Inc).

14
Getting on with Your Life: a User's Experience of Participating in the EMILIA Project

Torill Klevan Nilsen

My name is Torill Klevan Nilsen, and I was a user representative in the EMILIA project.

In February 2006, Mental Health in Bodø, a user organisation of which I am a member, was contacted regarding providing a user representative for an EU project. The project was called EMILIA. Asked to participate, I joined the project in mid-February 2006. I was somewhat frightened, somewhat confused and not sure if I could do this. The fact that all written material was in a foreign language (English) was a challenge in itself. Expressions such as *lifelong learning* and *empowerment* were buzzing in the air. Everything was new, and nothing made sense to me. It was also not clear to me as to what was expected of me as a user representative, or what predefined role I was to have. However, I decided to give myself, and the project, some time, allow myself to wait on the sidelines to see whether things became clearer with time.

So I clung on, and gradually I saw the contours of a project that in time would be of great significance to me personally, and hopefully to other users as well. My first encounter with other participants in EMILIA was at a meeting in Barcelona in October 2006. To be given the opportunity to participate in the annual meeting was an accomplishment in itself. Clearly, there was no longstanding tradition for the involvement of users. Realising I was the only user representative present, I felt both disappointment and frustration. The table was encircled by professionals, determining what users needed. Lifelong learning can be a lot of different things. I believe that the project itself had to learn how to allow users to participate to a greater extent, starting at the planning stage. There is a kind of arrogance to a project emphasising user participation that takes so long to involve users. But, change in thought and action does take time: in this instance, for both the users in the project and for those responsible for the project. As a professional, you have to dare and let some of your authority go, and as a user you have to let go some of the security that lies in passively accepting help. These are challenges for both parties.

Bodø was one of the demonstration sites in the project, and thus tested some of the training packages developed. The thought behind most training packages was that there should be two trainers, and that one of these was to have user experience. I was a trainer for two of the training packages in Bodø (Powerful Voices and Social Network Support). Cooperating with the other trainer, a professional, was a positive experience. Interacting with participants in the training packages felt meaningful and good. Based on my experience as a trainer, I have since taken part in a cooperative development of 'Interactive European Lifelong Learning Programmes' between Århus (Denmark) and Bodø, where I have experienced what I would term 'real user influence'. I define real user influence as participating on equal terms as other group members, where the divide between users and others is nonexistent. The focal point is how you can contribute, not who you are.

At several occasions I have contributed in presentations of the project within Norway, where I have talked about the project from a user's perspective. There seems to have been an increasing interest in EMILIA, and I would have to say my personal belief in the importance of the project has grown over time. I have personally experienced the importance of learning in secure surroundings. I had a hard time finding such safe surroundings when I needed them. Either expectations of users would be overwhelming, as in the municipal programmes; or there would be neither expectations nor demands, as in the psychiatric healthcare programmes. EMILIA offered the combination of safety and demands I was looking for.

The impact of the EMILIA project

When talking about change and to what degree change has taken place, one has to take a step back. It is when looking back that I realise what change has taken place. When the process was actually taking place, being present in the moment was more than sufficient.

My participation in EMILIA was based on my experiences of being mentally ill. It was this special competence as a user that was in demand. When asked to participate in the project in February 2006, my life situation was different than it is now. I had only recently embarked on the journey returning to a meaningful life, not sure where the road would take me. In 1990, my life had changed dramatically. I was 40 years old, married and the mother of two children. I worked full time and was actively involved in the community, in addition to being a mother and housewife. I lived what you might call a normal life, apparently successful. Deep down I had known for a long time that something was not right, that I carried a baggage from early years filled with traumatic experiences. I had spent a lot of energy keeping those memories at a distance through the years. In 1990, I hit the wall, the dam burst and I went down.

The following ten years felt as if I was moving through a dark emptiness. I had previously thought of myself as a sensible, able human being, independent in almost everything. Suddenly, I found myself dependent in most things. I gave up on life. My goal was to end it. Finding an end to life was my project for years. I lived through an existential void, an absence of life, abandoned by both people and God. Keeping up an existence in this void was not possible and I realised that if I chose life, I had to 'find life' somewhere. I had to venture into the world and dare take part in it. I was lucky. I had some good people around me, who had faithfully been there through all those years, who never gave up on me, who saw my strengths and not only my weaknesses. They believed in me, and with their help, and as others joined in, I embarked on the long road back to life. It was a strenuous process. I had lost so much over those years. I had gotten a divorce and moved out on my own. I left the workforce, and became a receiver of disability pension. Thus, my personal finances had taken a turn for the worse. I had isolated myself socially for long periods at a time. I suffered from a lack of concentration, and even reading became difficult – a big sorrow for a book-lover like me. Not the least, I had lost all self-confidence and self-esteem. As a human being, I was worthless, unsure of deserving to live.

Put simply, it was no easy task I had before me, but I had started and was well on way when I joined EMILIA.

What has EMILIA done for me, and where am I today?

A lot has happened in my life the past four years, events that have shaped my life, encounters with people of great significance. Isolating the factors making a difference is no easy task. Was one event more significant than another? It may be a mix of everything. But I do know that my involvement with EMILIA has been of great significance to me, and that I would not have been where I am today without EMILIA. The word 'recovery' has become particularly meaningful to me, it is a suitable equivalent for what has happened to me over these last years.

When I first joined this project, I encountered some unfamiliar terms for which I had to spend a fair amount of time to find understandable definitions and good Norwegian translations. The latter has been a challenge, and there is a tendency to use the English expressions in Norway. What first comes to mind is 'empowerment' and 'lifelong learning', both key terms in EMILIA.

For me, 'empowerment' consists both of using one's potential and neutralising what is hindering one in using one's potential. In my mind, empowerment cannot be given to a person, it is a want that has to come from within. Surroundings can help fight harassment, stigmatisation or neglect, and thus make it somewhat easier. But each individual has to clear his or her own path. My challenge then was realising what was holding me back from using my skills and abilities. Could I as an adult age dare use myself, believe in myself? To achieve this I needed arenas where I could challenge myself. My participation in EMILIA became one such arena.

Ever since I first became a user representative in EMILIA, I have been met with respect, and taken seriously. I do not think I will ever forget the moment when I was invited to join the annual meeting in Barcelona. It was for me a great honour and a real self-confidence boost, both personally and as a user representative. From a state of social and professional isolation, I had suddenly become part of a community. I had things to talk about, experiences to share. Life became richer in so many ways. I almost felt 'normal'. With the same obviousness I was invited to Barcelona, where I was given tasks and relied on to such a degree that it initially scared me, but I chose to believe I was capable. To be given the role as a trainer was a new and incredibly rewarding experience. I may have wished I had more knowledge and training, but I did OK. Cooperating with the professional trainer was very positive; I perceived we were a team. I got to use facets of myself besides those of a user, something that also gave a boost to my self-confidence. Working with course participants was a real source of motivation.

In what way can I relate lifelong learning to my personal experiences from participating in EMILIA, and what significance has it had on who I am today?

To be given the opportunity to visit other countries, to have a glimpse of other cultures and to hear foreign languages, has both been informative and of importance to me in social settings. I have gained knowledge and experiences that I can share with others. I have been given the opportunity to actively use a foreign language, English, to an extent I would never have achieved without participating in the project. This has been a real benefit to me. Old knowledge I thought long gone has come back to me: another self-confidence boost.

After years of social isolation, being forced to cooperate closely with others and also to function socially have been a learning experience and a demanding process. This may be where I have noticed the greatest change in myself. I have on several occasions been required to deliver written materials, which has led to a rediscovery of old computer skills, and the acquisition of new skills within the context of the ever-changing digital world. This has all been really inspiring.

The examples mentioned above are visible, tangible results of learning. Less tangible but so important is the impact of learning on the heart and mind, the challenges, not visible to anyone else, encountered and conquered, the anxiety I have had to combat to move on to experience personal growth. I have gained confidence in myself. I have found the courage to face new challenges, the courage to try and to fail. I have found courage to demand my space, to be more visible. I have allowed myself to dream, and to realise some of my dreams. Last fall, I went back to school to realise an old dream. I studied history of philosophy and could experience the joy of learning, the gratefulness of improved concentration and with that improved memory.

I have more dreams, and I will not abandon them. I will remember EMILIA as much more than a project. Through EMILIA, I was given a new beginning. I have been being relied on, something that has made me believe in myself and led me today to have a meaningful life. From this point on, it all depends on me.

15
Service Users' Experiences of Lifelong Learning

Irja Nieminen, Torill Klevan Nilsen, Isard Vila, María Trinidad Solá and the Fenix users group

This chapter is based on interviews with 23 users of mental health services who were members of the EMILIA project between 2007 and 2010. They were interviewed when they joined the project, at 10-month follow up and 20-month follow up. Overall, lifelong learning and the project as a whole were perceived as being a positive experience. The EMILIA training provided a stimulating challenge for mental health service users, gave them useful information and skills, and increased their social networks. Through the EMILIA training, they gained insight into lifelong learning. They understood that '*not all knowledge comes from books*' and that they had already learnt many things during their lives. Findings in this chapter concur with the observation that learning does not happen only at schools, within an official teaching system, but also includes individual and social learning in all surroundings, formally at schools and non-formally at home, at work and in the community (Eurydice European Unit 2000).

Experiences of learning: empowerment and social inclusion

Learning with other people and forming relationships with those who share similar experiences are perceived to be valuable in terms of recovery and as a mental health protective factor by mental health service users (Clayton and Tse 2003, Hammond 2004). Participation in a group builds social self-confidence; increased self-esteem and independence impact positively on the ability of individuals to cope with potentially difficult situations (Hammond 2004). In EMILIA, participating in the group was initially experienced as being a difficult process. As one EMILIA user stated, it was 'particularly important to be able to sit in the group, listen to a trainer, and ask questions without being judged as being weird'. They had to learn to work in a group, to be with others and to share tasks. Group work was an important experience, as they discovered that their ideas can be conveyed to others in a way understood by others. This made them feel recognised, understood and validated their sense of self. The opportunity to help others as a result of learning was a big boost to self-confidence.

Being in the EMILIA training also meant finding out that there are others in a similar situation with regard to being mental ill. Participating in EMILIA provided a purpose in life and helped participants feel more positive; coming to the training every week gave a sense of stability. EMILIA was perceived as enabling personal growth in finding one's own strengths and acquiring more insight about oneself. Some attributes, before perceived by service users to be weaknesses, were now trans-formed into being seen as strengths. Self-confidence increased and users found they had the courage to do new things. One of the users described his experiences of how he overcame his fear and was able to teach others; his confidence in his ability to learn and teach despite of his mental illness increased substantially:

> My friend was enrolled in my group where we were learning to make costume jewellery. I showed him how to make a necklace and he was happy. I was satisfied with meeting him. I was satisfied in overcom-ing my fear. I was satisfied in having the opportunity to show the patients in the hospital everything I can do and to show to the doc-tors that regardless of my illness I am able to learn, I can show what I have learned to others, and that I can adequately leave the psychi-atric hospital. This was an experience that I will never ever forget.

Users felt they had learned to become more responsible for their own treatment; they had more tools for recovery, and had learned to live with their illness better. Participating in the EMILIA training gave users the experience of being listened to and being treated as equals. They were not seen only as mental health patients, but holistically as multi-layered people, and hence felt respected.

Learning of course also enabled mental health service users to gain new skills and knowledge (Isenwater, Lanham and Thornhill 2002, Barnes, Carpenter and Dickinson 2006, Ramon et al. 2011). They are motivated to find jobs and learning new skills is a step in this direc-tion (Secker, Grove and Seebohm 2001), reducing financial dependence and improving quality of life (Megivern, Pellerito and Mowbray 2003). In EMILIA, users from Bosnia described their experience of the lifelong learning programme and how they gained new skills through which they were able to train others. Access to lifelong learning was a largely new experience:

> Enrolment of our user group in the lifelong learning programme at the very beginning seemed very strange and unknown to us. Our first meeting with people who came to show to us something that we can learn and from which we can maybe gain some profit felt surprisingly good. We knew there was no chance or possibility to be offered a job in a company. With our diagnoses, we could expect simply to be on long-term sick leave until retirement. Retirement benefits were not sufficient, and days without work made us more depressive and withdrawn. We felt even more worthless and useless.

Learning practical skills (in Bosnia) opened up new horizons.

> Firstly we learnt how to make jewellery. When the first ring, necklace, earring or bracelets were made, we found out that they were nice and attracted the attention and interest of others, which aroused our enthusiasm. When we learned that people wanted to buy what we make, our enthusiasm was special. This way we started to earn money for material and to make new things. We stopped asking local authorities to provide us money for material, because we could do it on our own. Then we learned vase and glass modelling: working with glass, making coasters and many small household things.

Acquiring skills and employment increased self-esteem, which in turn brought new ideas.

> Our self-confidence has increased. We were of importance to ourselves and others. We showed these things to our friends. The most interesting is that we learned all this in the group and helping each other. Working with trainers, we got the idea to redo our courtyard where we used to spend plenty of time. Then we made a fireplace and a tree shelter in the yard. We found unusual tree stumps in the woods and brought them there. We made stone mosaics on the grass and our courtyard became a big workshop with many interesting things which attracted attention in our surroundings.

The local community became interested in what they were doing.

It helped us to become interesting to our neighbours, our street, and our society. They did not turn their eyes away; they started coming to our courtyard, being interested in our work, asking us to arrange their courtyards the same way we did it with our yard. Then we were offered a job by our first neighbour and we have arranged his yard. He was very satisfied. Learning to make costume jewellery, small home decorations, kitchen things, ties and glass work, contributed to our initiative asking our municipality to support us in opening a cooperative where we could make these things and sell them with the aim of self-financing our Association and providing financial support for those who would work there. For us, learning is always possible; there is no obstacle for learning due to illness or age.

In Denmark, some of the users who participated in the EMILIA project underwent training to become Personal Medicine Coaches (PMC). The training was structured around themes such as medication, active listening, coping strategies and recovery. After training, the PMCs coached service users who wish to receive guidance from a peer with special skills and lived experience in this field.

The fact that EMILIA was being carried out in different places in Europe was also motivating. Users appreciated the fact that similar training packages were being implemented in seven other sites around Europe. They clearly saw some of the topics of the training, notably stigma, as transcultural. One user remarked: '*The idea of living in a community but not being part of it is something patients like me could understand anywhere*'. The forming of not just a local EMILIA group but a greater European one was regarded as prestigious and worked as a booster to their confidence. One user aptly expressed herself by saying: '*I feel that I'm being recognized as a European citizen*'.

Research shows that students benefit from being on a course with other users and ex-users of mental health services (Isenwater, Lanham and Thornhill 2002). Peer-support and support from the lecturers are crucial factors in improving functioning within and outside college (Hammond 2004). Having social support is also one of the most important things which help mental health service users to succeed in their education (Bybee, Bellamy and Mowbray 2000, Collins, Mowbray and Bybee 2000, Tinklin, Riddell and Wilson 2005, Padron 2006). In EMILIA, sharing knowledge and experience, learning in a peer group allowing all participants to contribute was felt to be a good learning situation. Users in the EMILIA training considered that good and open communication, having time to talk and listen, as well as having regular meetings, facilitated learning. The training packages for users created a space where users felt safe to ask questions and share experiences. One user commented on the freedom the EMILIA training had given him, by which he meant finding a group of people who understood him and did not judge him. Others spoke about how they appreciated the fact that they were 'taken seriously'. Experiencing safety, unity and solidarity in the group was found to be important in the EMILIA training. Easy access to training helped users to participate in training more readily.

Experiences as trainers

Individuals with a mental illness have much to contribute in terms of knowledge about the specificities of mental illness and its effects. Education involving tutoring also enables users to reap personal benefits such as learning new skills, increased self-confidence and a genuine feeling of empowerment (Masters et al. 2002). They can also act as role models for other service users, as they offer personal examples of the potential to overcome the limitations imposed by the experience of the illness, and can use this experience to help others. As the EMILIA project developed, a growing number of users worked as trainers. The fact that users could and should be trainers not only for other users, but for mental health care professionals as well, promoted recovery. Users began to value their knowledge as patients and saw how they could build upon their experiences as users of mental health services. One of the users described her own experiences as a trainer, how she could use her experiences of being mentally ill as an important element of her competence:

> As a user representative in the EMILIA steering group in our site, my main task was to focus on the user perspective. That meant the competence which was asked for was my experience derived from being mentally ill. It was a special competence which I could contribute with. I have thought about this a bit: although I would rather not have had the experience of being mentally ill, it felt OK that it could be used in a constructive way. This was something I had knowledge of and that someone wanted to listen to. This did something to the way I saw myself. I experienced that I was actually being taken seriously, that I had something to contribute.

By working as a trainer, she learnt new skills and also found her past, forgotten skills. Training others was a learning situation in itself, another part of lifelong learning.

Obstacles to learning

The symptoms of mental illness can make it difficult to concentrate, remember and keep up motivation (Megivern, Pellerito and Mowbray 2003) and reduce the ability to stand stress (Secker, Grove and Seebohm 2001), thus leading certain learners to interrupt participation in learning situations (Megivern, Pellerito and Mowbray 2003). Experiencing mental distress impacts on the ability to participate in social activities (Padron 2006) and the ability to communicate (Ryan, Woodyatt and Copeland. 2010), thus also impeding social inclusion. For some users in EMILIA, the mental illness itself, stress, personal shortcomings, low self-confidence, difficulty to get to the sessions or personality clashes with fellow participants or teachers, made learning difficult. Some found it difficult to understand the meaning of certain training themes. Training sessions were sometimes felt to be too long. Some participants were skeptical about mental health service users taking part in training, whereas others had expectations that were sometimes too high. Users said that these attitudes prevented their learning.

Discrimination and stigma are major obstacles to mental health service users' social inclusion and access to employment. A service user in Tuzla described this situation:

> With regard to employment, the only problem I faced was to get a health certificate (to demonstrate) that I am capable for work. Our association considered me as capable, while doctors thought that I could not do it. Plenty of time was needed to convince the doctors to issue a medical approval for me for the position of a workshop leader. I was not the only one with this problem. One much younger friend of mine who was supposed to get a secretary job within the association had the same problem. In our self-help group, we discussed the problem of getting medical approval for work. Regardless of being capable to work or have skills, when a person is diagnosed with schizophrenia, doctors who consider that schizophrenic people will never be able to work become an obstacle.

Another user described her experiences of stigma and prejudice after becoming mentally ill and how she began to feel being excluded from society:

> There is still a lot of stigma and prejudice connected to mental illnesses. I experienced that at one time people around me had

stopped asking things of me, expected nothing of me, and had stopped believing in me. I was sick and that was it. Just as if I stopped being an individual. This did something to me, I began to believe them, that they were right and that I wasn't 'useable'.

The service-user group in Tuzla in Bosnia had to face a double stigma firstly because of their mental ill health and secondly because being unemployed is a condition for receiving their war pension. They were entitled to invalidity benefits due to traumatic experiences they had had during the war in Yugoslavia (1992–5), but to require them by law not to work only added to that trauma.

Conclusion

Mental health service users in the EMILIA Project consider lifelong learning as useful and it improves their quality of life in many ways. Learning gives improved knowledge and skills, a better social life, stronger self-confidence and a possibility to be employed. All of these areas are extremely important concerning not only lifelong learning but also social inclusion. Users felt that they are marked by mental illness, in the sense that stigma and discrimination against people with mental illness in society still operate, impeding their learning and social inclusion. However, during the EMILIA project, users were able to feel more socially included. They were able to find their own strength and to build upon it. The realization that all knowledge does not come from formal education helped them to value their own knowledge and experiences as mental health service users. The knowledge gained from their own experiences and those of fellow service users about being a patient was – and is – valuable for both other people with mental illness and especially for mental health professionals.

References

Barnes, D., Carpenter, J. and Dickinson, C. (2006). 'The Outcomes of Partnerships with Mental Health Service Users in Interprofessional Education: A Case Study', *Health and Social Care in the Community*, XIV, 426–35.
Bybee, D., Bellamy, C. and Mowbray, C. T. (2000). 'Analysis of Participation in an Innovative Psychiatric Rehabilitation Intervention: Supported Education', *Evaluation and Program Planning*, XXIII, 41–52.
Clayton, J. and Tse, S. (2003). 'An Educational Journey Towards Recovery for Individuals with Persistent Mental Illnesses: A New Zealand Perspective', *Psychiatric Rehabilitation Journal*, XXVII, 72–8.

Collins, M. E., Mowbray, C. T. and Bybee, D. (2000). 'Characteristics Predicting Successful Outcomes of Participants with Severe Mental Illness in Supported education', *Psychiatric Services*, LI, 774–80.

Eurydice European Unit (2000). 'Lifelong Learning: The Contribution of Education Systems in the Member States of the European Union Results of the EURYDICE Survey', http://www.mp.gov.rs/resursi/dokumenti/dok81-eng-LLL.2.pdf, date accessed 28 December 2011.

Hammond, C. (2004). 'Impacts of Lifelong Learning upon Emotional Resilience, Psychological and Mental Health: Fieldwork Evidence', *Oxford Review of Education* XXX, 551–68.

Isenwater, W., Lanham, W. and Thornhill, H. (2002). 'The College Link Program: Evaluation of a Supported Education Initiative in Great Britain', *Psychiatric Rehabilitation Journal* XXVI, 43–50.

Masters, H., Forrest, S., Harley, A., Hunter, M., Brown, N. and Risk, I. (2002). 'Involving Mental Health Service Users and Carers in Curriculum Development: Moving Beyond 'Classroom' Involvement', *Journal of Psychiatric and Mental Health Nursing* IX, 309–16.

Megivern, D., Pellerito, S. and Mowbray, C. (2003). 'Barriers to Higher Education for Individuals with Psychiatric Disabilities', *Psychiatric Rehabilitation Journal* XXVI, 217–31.

Padron, J. M. (2006). 'Experience with Post-Secondary Education for Individuals with Severe Mental Illness', *Psychiatric Rehabilitation Journal* XXX, 147–9.

Ramon, S., Griffiths, C. A., Nieminen, I., Pedersen, M. L. and Dawson, I. (2011). 'Towards Social Inclusion through Lifelong Learning in Mental Health: Analysis of Change in the Lives of the EMILIA Project Service Users', *International Journal of Social Psychiatry* LVII, 211–23.

Ryan, J., Woodyatt, G. and Copeland, D. (2010). 'Procedural Discourse in Intellectual Disability and Dual Diagnosis', *Journal of Intellectual Disability Research* LIV, 70–80.

Secker, J., Grove, B. and Seebohm, P. (2001). 'Challenging Barriers to Employment, Training and Education for Mental Health Service Users: The Service User's Perspective', *Journal of Mental Health* X, 395–404.

Tinklin, T., Riddell, S. and Wilson, A. (2005). 'Support for Students with Mental Health Difficulties in Higher Education: The Students' Perspective', *British Journal of Guidance & Counselling* XXXIII, 495–512.

16
Mental Health Service Users as Trainers in the Context of the EMILIA Project

Terese Stenfors-Hayes and Peter Ryan

Introduction

Lifelong learning is a basic component of the European social model; however, adult learning is the weak link in the lifelong learning framework and there is an increasing recognition around Europe that a fundamentally new approach to education policies should be developed (COM 2001). Educational systems need to be made more flexible and more accessible to a wider range of people (Schleicher 2006). To achieve this, many of the world's most successful educational systems have shifted focus from uniformity in their system to one that embraces diversity and individualised learning (Schleicher 2006). EU documents have mentioned tailoring learning opportunities to individual citizens as part of the strategy to achieve social cohesion and employment (COM 2001 and OECD 2005), but more progress is required to apply these proclamations to groups such as those with mental health problems.

Policy-makers recognise that because particular groups are socially excluded and that they can be difficult to reach, assertive measures are required to be able to offer them lifelong learning opportunities. However, relatively little has been done to identify creative ways to include socially excluded groups such as those with long-term mental health difficulties. This is an area where EMILIA has been very innovative and where the project has learnt a great deal, in particular the strategic importance of peer to peer learning through sharing experiences: using service users as trainers was a very productive and valuable part of the approach to lifelong learning as adopted in the EMILIA project.

Through sharing experiences, individuals can learn beyond the actual content of the modules; this social interaction is of a supportive nature and encourages cohesion in the learning group. This approach to learning is sometimes referred to as PAL (peer assisted learning): with 'people from similar social groupings who are not professional teachers helping each other to learn and learning themselves by so doing' (Topping 1996). This provides opportunity for learners to learn in a small, friendly group thereby co-creating a collaborative learning environment. Ross and Cumming (2005) list a number of advantages for PAL tutoring that easily can be related to the approaches undertaken in the EMILIA project:

• provides opportunities to reinforce and revise learning
• encourages responsibility and increased self-confidence
• enhances communication skills, empathy and self-appraisal skills
• encourages reflection and self-direction
• enhances organisational and team working skills

By learning to teach, the learner also learns to learn by recognising learning processes in their peers. This will sharpen their meta-cognitive skills (Biggs 1999). Peer teaching also supports improvement of social skills and attitudes to study and self (Biggs 1999). Teaching is by many believed to be the best way to learn but a PAL approach does not need to be used only in formal learning, it works equally well in informal or non formal settings. Being taught by a peer is also beneficial from a learning perspective: the atmosphere is usually more relaxed, many opportunities for feedback are usually given, peers usually find it easy to understand each other, and people may be less hesitant to ask questions.

In this chapter, a Learning and Teaching Model developed by Ross and Stenfors-Hayes (2008) will be used to describe what service-user trainers in the EMILIA project did and how aspects such as the trainer personality and the situation affected the training. The interviews focused on what it had meant to them to be trainers, and if and how this had affected their lives especially in terms of learning and empowerment. In the chapter, perspectives from EMILIA trainers with no mental health service-user background will also be included as well as the service user as student perspective.

The learning and teaching model (see Figure 16.1)

The learning and teaching model focuses on an individual **Learner** and **Teacher** and the interactions between them. Both learner and teacher have their own personality, prior experience, knowledge, skills,

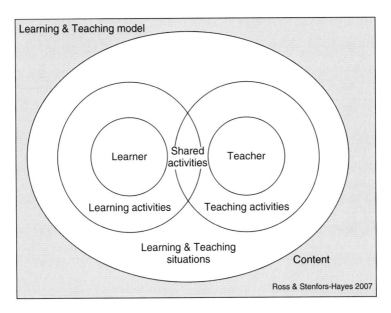

Figure 16.1 Learning and teaching model

attitudes and other commitments which may impact upon the learner's learning. The model is a simplification in which there may be parallel interactions between multiple learners and teachers and others, and in which assignment of these roles may not remain static (the teacher may become the learner and vice-versa). Learner and teacher engage respectively in **Learning Activities** and **Teaching Activities** – purposeful activities aimed at enabling the learner to learn. Most activities are not done together, although **Shared Activities** involve some dialogue or transaction, either face-to-face or at a distance. All activities take place in **Learning & Teaching Situations**. These can be described by variables such as physical location (class room, library, home) or numbers present (individual, small group and large group teaching). In these situations, learner and teacher engage with **Content**. In this chapter, the model is also used as a framework to analyse qualitative data gathered from EMILIA service-user trainers undertaking lifelong learning training in the eight demonstration sites of the EMILIA project.

Within the EMILIA project, the training produced and offered has been evaluated mainly through feedback from students. The training packages referred to are available online (emiliatraining.net) and have been available to all people involved throughout the whole project.

Method

All eight demonstration sites were contacted and a list of all English-speaking trainers and producers of the training packages was put together. Trainers and training material producers were subsequently contacted by the first author and interviewed using video conference equipment if available, via telephone or face-to face. Altogether, nine trainers and three training material producers and/or supporting trainers were interviewed. The supporting trainers were university staff attending the training run by EMILIA participants. The trainers had in these cases planned and developed the training in collaboration with the supporting trainers but ran the sessions on their own. The interviews were recorded and transcribed. After a first reading of all the transcripts, it was decided that the teaching and learning model would be used as a tool and framework for the analysis and the description of the training.

Findings and analysis

The EMILIA students

All students taking the EMILIA training were mental health service users with a diagnosis of schizophrenia or bi-polar disorder, with at least five years experience of receiving mental health services, and all were currently unemployed.

The findings from the interviews are presented according to the different sections of the learning and teaching model, in the following order:

- content
- learning and teaching situations
- shared activities
- teaching activities
- the teacher
- learning activities

Content

The EMILIA training has been based on different modules such as 'strengths', 'research' and 'social networks'. But the interviews showed that the content might still have varied significantly within these different modules. The content of the courses in many places seem to have been developed over time and within the shared learning group. Often there was considerable emphasis on tailoring the training material as originally specified to the local situation and to local training needs:

> We revamped because we wanted it to be locally relevant. What we taught was actually very different from the original workshop.

The interview from which this first quote stems further describes what a roller coaster it was to be a trainer, how he/she went in to the classroom armed with ideas and exercises but in reality had no idea where he/she would end up, where the group would take him/her.

> The purpose of the programmes was to get the experience they had and to share it. They learnt nothing new but rather became aware of what they already knew.

A lot of the training has been focused on bringing out already existing knowledge and skills, rather than imposing new one's.

> Hope is the central theme, if there is just a little bit of light, I hope we've made it a little bit lighter.

The themes that keep reoccurring such as hope, empowerment, and strengths offer another way of looking at the data. The interviews showed that the themes that flow through the courses and the dynamic process through which the content was developed, is what signified the content of the EMILIA training.

> It's not just hope it's also opportunity that we need to provide.

Another aspect is the connection between the course and the 'real world' as the last quote shows. In this case, this relates to employment and work opportunities.

Learning and teaching situations

When describing a learning and teaching situation, the discussion commonly focuses on aspects such as virtual or face to face, degree of formality, or the number of learners. However, in this study, we found there were two main aspects of the situation: the physical aspects of the room and the location (practicalities), as well as the emotional aspects.

Practicalities

The location of the room, sometimes in a university and sometimes in a hospital, varied and this might have some importance. Also the exact location of the room was discussed a lot, for example the possibility to go outside easily or not, being in the middle of a big campus, which some participants might have found intimidating. Time and length varied a lot at the different demonstration sites, but all seem to have worked well in their particular case. Some had afternoons, some whole days; what they all have shared is the social side, where meals are included and perhaps the coffee breaks were not really breaks, but just another aspect of the experience. Many also mentioned that it is important to make time to take medication and keep doctor's appointments. What was found most central here was the possibility to influence the situation, with the users participating in designing the training then and there (not necessarily just before), including the possibility of leaving or speaking privately with a trainer for support.

Emotional aspects: feeling safe

The first emotional aspect of the training was feeling safe: 'it is a grey zone between public and private so you need to feel safe and secure in order to be able to talk about these things.' Equality in the group and between trainers and students and trainers and demonstration site staff was frequently discussed and relates to the theme of being able to influence the training, and feeling that your own opinion counts and will be listened to. The training was also described as being moving, powerful and personal 'It was very powerful and also sharing that with so many other people who were also on their own journeys was very powerful'.

Shared activities

The training seems to have been very process oriented. A lot of time was taken to 'settle into' the training, establish how people were feeling that particular day, if they were okay to be there and what was happening to them at that moment. Both trainers and learners shared their personal experiences and feelings and they reflected upon these together. Some trainers, who were used to teaching in different, more formal contexts, described this as somewhat new to them; they were not used to training being so personal. Although this is why feeling safe was so important, but sometimes it may be difficult to draw the line for what to share and not so share. The social aspects of the training (breaks, meals...) were also frequently brought up, and also social activities outside the organised training such as going out to a restaurant together after the training had finished, or going to a culture event together. The classroom activities were very varied and included: lectures, presentations, big group, small group, buzz groups, role play, hands-on exercises, story telling, music, real cases, questionnaires, drawing and homework groups. Again, all of these were very much adapted to the group, some started maybe with a particular concept to discuss or an article and other exercises were very hands on, including smashing eggs or papaya, as a palpable symbol of the potential fragility of service users themselves. Some worked with real everyday situations from the hospital. Many trainers described how surprised they were to see how much time the exercises and the training took. As they became more experienced trainers, they included less content in the programme, allowing more and more time for discussion and reflection.

Teaching activities

The teaching activities are presented and grouped into three different themes, using the model proposed by Ross and Stenfors-Hayes (2008).

1. *Facilitating learning*
   This theme includes creating an opportunity to learn, through motivation and minimising barriers: encouragement, trying to ignite something, listen to the students, bring out existing knowledge and experiences to build upon. This theme also includes role modelling, sharing their own experiences and challenging, and provoking.
2. *Managing learning*
   This theme includes leading the classroom process, trying to gently move some discussions forward, but at the same time making sure everyone is feeling that they can speak up. It seems to have been a quite common problem to keep the right 'speed' and not dwell. Also having support available if a student experienced an emotional crisis; a participant might be reminded of a previous trauma and need individual support or a short break for example. Another aspect of managing learning was persuading people to come and arranging transport if necessary. Inviting other trainers or experts to participate and introducing learners as trainers was also included in this theme. Session and course organisation and development were also part of this theme. Evaluation together with peer teachers, and participants

was done in different ways in different sites. Also making sure there was not too much overlap between different courses. The trainers also used their own experiences when planning the teaching. Some talked about how they liked to learn themselves and planned the training according to that.

3. *Learning and Community Building*

    Informal reflective practice and learning for the trainers was also part of the EMILIA training experience as many trainers also learnt a lot about the actual classroom process and leading discussions. Respondents who lacked user experience themselves all mentioned how much they learnt about being a user and from working with users, and people that have taught before talk about a new way of working; many of them have never worked this closely together with the learners before. One respondent said it had also had an impact on their clinical practice. Many of them mentioned how being a trainer has spurred them to learn more, take a teacher training course, study a particular topic or similar. Community building in the form of user advisory groups or training new trainers is also part of this theme as well as collaboration and networking within EMILIA and for some this has lead to other opportunities outside of EMILIA in terms of presenting their experiences and teaching in other contexts.

The teacher

Who the trainer is and his or her previous knowledge and experience also affect the training and the students' learning. What was seen in these interviews is that the trainers often structure the training based on how they themselves like to learn and their own experiences:

> You have to know your topic, be aware of the process and guide and assist in what is going on in the room equally as much as you deliver your material.

This is another example of how the trainers 'use themselves' in the training. Naturally, they also have expertise in different fields, some more medical, others in facilitating personal development, and so on. Sometimes trainers with or without user experience working together seem to have taken on slightly different roles and some trainers claimed that the participants came to them with different questions, depending on their background. Some trainers with user experience felt that they could 'put more pressure' on the students and challenge them more, while trainers without this background may contribute more with expertise from a certain theoretical field. User experience was also a way to legitimise the training.

What should the teacher be like? Capable of containing a lot of people with very different needs and personalities.

This quote describes what a trainer should be like. According to our analysis it seems like it has a lot to do with a certain generosity of spirit, being able to accept people in all their variability and vulnerability, without judgement or criticism. It also implies being generous with your own experiences and also generous with inviting people to create the course with you and let them take up the emotional space which they need.

Learning activities

This part of the model may illustrate one of the most significant differences from the context where this model was originally developed in. For undergraduate medical students, only a small part is what they do together in a group context, while they study a lot at home, in clinical wards, and so on. In EMILIA, the shared activities are more central, which probably relates to the social aspect of the training and to coming to training from a very different perspective, being interested in how the training can support the trainees in a holistic way, rather than focusing only on providing knowledge and skills. For example, when the trainers realised at one demonstration site that it did not work particularly well with asking the students to do homework on their own, so instead they provided time and place for them to come in a do it together. (While in higher education today many students do not even come to the University Lectures or seminars, but follow them online instead.)

The learners

The trainers also talked about how the students identified their already existing knowledge, which sometimes could take some time. There are also some other consequences of the training such as a learner inviting friends home for a meal for the first time.

There is a transformation in some of the students...
You saw that they grew!

One aspect of the learner is how they were viewed by the trainers. One trainer pointed out that it is important to let them be students and to view them as students, not just mental health service users. Others also mentioned that this was a completely new target group; previously they had thought they were too ill. Some examples of aspects that the trainers felt that they needed to take into consideration when they planned the training was: motivation and learning needs, previous experiences of all kinds (including traumas), attention span, stress tolerance level, diagnosis or level of functioning.

The service user as student

The data described in this section is drawn from the 3-5 key informant interviews which were conducted in each of the eight demonstration sites.

Some respondents claimed that the training had meant a lot to them: it gave some a sense of meaning to life. Another respondent described it as an improved quality of life and for some it meant personal growth.

> As I've already said, on several occasions, any education is good education, if in addition you meet nice people and share and exchange experience and ideas with them, then, well, you're richer spiritually. You grow.

It has also meant improved self confidence, realisation of own skills and strengths and motivation and knowledge about their illness and how to try and overcome it and recovery mechanisms.

> It motivated me – I found a job.

The friendship and contact with other people was also very meaningful as well as the support given. Some respondents felt recognised for their skills and strengths.

> Contact with people who have the same problems empowers, it makes me believe that something can be done.

> Professionals believed we have abilities, strengths, I finally felt good about myself.

Many respondents believed they had improved their communication skills and were proud to be able to do a public presentation. Some had also realised how useful their experiences could be and that they can be used to help others and themselves.

I can use my experience to help myself and others.

Learning in EMILIA was motivated by the high involvement and level of interaction in the training. The level of motivation varied however, some were very motivated while other respondents struggled with *depression* and therefore found it difficult to appreciate the training.

Factors in the EMILIA training that facilitated learning

The good communication between participants and trainers is the most commonly mentioned facilitating factor. The patience of trainers is also a reoccurring theme.

> They were really patient with us, well not with me, I'm good, but with some members who are not very artistic.
> We can repeat things, and ask for clarification if we don't know how to use the glue.

The respectfulness of the trainers and the style and way in which they presented things were also mentioned and the feeling of being equal.

> We're all friends here, all equal.

In some demonstration sites, the training was delivered by service-user peers, which was appreciated and claimed to facilitate learning. Good communication also helped to develop a good atmosphere in the classroom.

> Well, it has given me the space in a relaxed and supportive atmosphere to learn, to really share and interact with colleges. So, yeah, that has been what it has been: a good space.

The informality of the situation was also appreciated. Some respondents acknowledged the opportunity to meet others in a similar situation and to feel that they could also help others. Although difficult at first, being trusted with responsibility was found to be very helpful:

> I couldn't guide myself through life, how could I guide someone else? ... I felt good, useful, important... you start from something small and build up to it.

More specific examples that were given used role plays and working with setting goals for oneself. Another exercise that was mentioned is described below:

> It was very simple – we stood at a certain place in the room and he [trainer] said: everyone go to where you think you are now and where you were a little while ago, and it showed how much you had improved but you didn't [previously] realise [that you had improved]. Sometimes I think to myself that I don't feel so good, but then I think how I was a little while ago. Little things like that for example [help].

The EMILIA training was described as being different from their previous training experiences by its content which focused on self-recovery and empowerment.

> It concerned my health, my social functioning, functioning in my family and among friends, my autonomy, and my activity.

The good communication in the group and between the trainers and trainees were also found to be unique to EMILIA. One respondent felt that in EMILIA they worked together to change their lives and difficulties were respected.

> I didn't feel like a failure... I felt like I had something to offer.

Barriers to learning in EMILIA

Obstacles mentioned by the respondents are few, as motivation was generally high. Depression was one barrier and low self-confidence another. Other barriers mentioned were trainers' own short-comings and difficulties in coming to terms with them and stress. One respondent identified laziness as a barrier as he/she found it difficult to leave home, but he/she was also aware of the therapeutic effect of making the effort to go to the training. One respondent thought that the training sometimes 'went over her head' and the trainers spoke too much and one of the modules was found to be difficult by another respondent:

> I didn't like the strengths module. That was very hard.
> –You found it to be too much of a challenge?
> No, I just found it difficult.

Lifelong learning

The respondents were asked to define what the concept of lifelong learning meant to them:

It means continuous work on oneself, getting new skills.
Well, it is part of that road to recovery. You are learning about yourself. It is about learning and reinventing and trying to flourish in life.
I think that it is useful to keep on learning throughout your life, whatever you are doing.

Discussion and conclusions

EMILIA is an example of training which was open and inclusive of people not often participating in formal training, and it may be that the combination of formal, non formal and informal training in EMILIA worked well as an introduction to more formal training for the participants, as some now aim to move on to for example higher education. The students in EMILIA had varying backgrounds, some with university degrees and even PhDs and others without any such experience. These varying backgrounds do not seem to have posed any problems; possible explanations for this may be found in the content of the training being new to most students and very focused on the student themselves and their recovery. The shared experience of being mental health service users or the training being adjustable to each individual based on his/her needs is other likely explanations. In fact, as reported in the demonstration site questionnaire, some sites would like to be even more inclusive and allow for anyone with severe mental illness to participate in the training. Increased self-confidence and self-esteem were reported as a result of the training and most students claimed that EMILIA was indeed a very positive experience for them, and this positive learning experience may well trigger future participation in training.

The principles that underpin European lifelong learning are centrality of the learner, equal opportunities and the quality and relevance of the learning opportunities (COM 2001). The aims of lifelong learning in Europe are to build an inclusive society, to adjust the ways in which education and training is provided, ensure that people's skills and knowledge meet the demands and to encourage and equip people to participate in all spheres of modern public life (COM 2002).

Lifelong learning in Europe further aims to promote the development of knowledge that helps people adapt to the knowledge-based society and take more control over their future. Formal, non-formal and informal learning are all valued and the learning pathway should be adjusted to each person's needs and interests in different stages of their life. The EMILIA training builds on these objectives and principles, and the empirical data presented in this chapter shows that these aims have been somewhat achieved. The EMILIA training has to a very large extent been adjusted to the students' needs and interests and the training has been perceived as equal and relevant. Furthermore, EMILIA included other socially inclusive parts of modern public life such as culture events and dinner at a restaurant for the students. The students describe plans for further training, some have got jobs, and others have increased their social circles.

Personal fulfilment is one of the key supporting objectives of lifelong learning (COM 2001). Instead of transmitting knowledge, the focus in European lifelong learning is on developing individual capabilities and personal learning competencies and at the centre of the concept of lifelong learning is the idea of encouraging and enabling people to learn how to learn (COM 2002). However, the EAEA (2006) claims that education with aims such as personal growth, increased self-esteem and social inclusion to a certain extent often is overlooked. In EMILIA, the focus has been on developing individual capabilities and bringing out already existing skills and knowledge. Many students plan to continue participating in training, for example in the Bonanova school in Barcelona or in higher education. This may imply that EMILIA has also helped the participants to learn how to learn, or at least encouraged them to learn.

References

Biggs, J. (1999). *Teaching for Quality learning at University* (Buckingham: SRHE & Open University Press).

COM (2001). *Making a European Area of Lifelong Learning*. European Commission. 678 Final. Brussels.

COM (2002). *A Memorandum on Lifelong Learning*. Commission staff working paper. Brussels. 1832.

EAEA (2006). Adult Education Trends and Issues in Europe. NO.EAC/43/05, Brussels.

OECD (2005). *Thematic Review on Adult Learning. Poland Country Note*. http://www.oecd.org, date accessed 14 June 2011.

Ross, M. T. and Cumming, A. D. (2005). 'Peer-Assisted Learning', in J. Dent and R. Harden (eds). *A Practical Guide for Medical Teachers* (Oxford: Elsevier).

Ross, M. T. and Stenfors-Hayes, T. (2008). 'Development of a Framework of Medical Undergraduate Teaching Activities', *Medical Education*, XLII, 915–22.

Schleicher, A. (2006). *The Economics of Knowledge: Why Education is Key for Europe's Success*. Lisbon Council Policy Brief, Brussels.

Topping, K. J. (1996). 'The Effectiveness of Peer Tutoring in Further and Higher Education: A Typology and Review of the Literature', *Studies in Higher Education*, XXXIII, 321–45.

Index

A

access to information and resources, 139, 152
accommodation, offering reasonable, 67
accountability of services, 152
active sense of self, 25
adequate supervision, providing, 67
advocacy, 167
agency, 71
alienation, 25
American Consumer Operated Services Program Multisite Research Initiative (COSP), 36
Americans with Disabilities Act, 95
Anderson, J., 154–67
Australia
mental health service reform in, 17
authorship, 24
avoidant coping style, 141

B

Bangkok Charter for Health Promotion in a Globalized World, 140
Barrett, R.J., 21, 142
barriers to people with mental illness
context, 112–14
obstacles and facilitators at the individual level, 114–15
obstacles and facilitators at the institutional level, 115–16
obstacles and facilitators at the macrosocial level, 116
Supported Employment Model
Basaglia, F., 92–4
Basset, T., 165
Becker, D.R.
on issues of Individual Placement and Support (IPS), 103–4
bipolar disorder F30-F31 (ICD-10), 120–1

Birleson, P., 194
blogs
for effective service-user involvement, 150
Bodø, 205
Bosnia
experience of service users in, 215
lifelong learning in, 176
Bosnia and Herzegovina –
lifelong learning in, 176
Brann, P., 194
broader community, policies focused on, 95–6
Brown, N., 105
'Building on Personal Strengths' training programme, 179

C

Campbell, K., 165
career aspirations, 115
Care Programme Approach (CPA), 55
Centre of Excellence in Interdisciplinary Mental Health (CEIMH), 159
Centres of Excellence in Teaching and Learning, 166
Chapman, V., 159
Charmaz, K., 185
clinically informed recovery, 23–4
cognitive impairment, 114
cognitive training, 114
Coldham, T., 162
collaborative learning initiatives, 162–3
community and mental health system, 92–4
community awareness in mental health systems, 92–6
community-based service systems, 88
community inclusion, 85–96, 92
overview, 85–7
policies focused on the mental health system, 87–92

policies for broader community, 95–6
policies for community awareness,
92–4
community integration, 85
community membership, 29
Complexity Theory approach, 193
connectedness, 25, 29, 138
Consultancy Development
Programme, 178
consumer perspective
on schizophrenia recovery, 23–4
contacts, 42
Copeland's five key principles of
recovery, 51
coping skills, 114
coping style, avoidant, 141
Crane-Ross
definition of service empowerment
by, 142
crisis plan, 53
Crosby, K., 159
Cy, M., 142–3

D
daily maintenance plan, 53
Danish conception of lifelong
learning, 176
data collection measures, 191
decision-making
inclusion in, 151–2
power, 138–9
Deegan, P.E., 180
Democratic Psychiatry movement, 92
demonstration sites, 79
Denmark
EMILIA project in, 212
depression, 141, 142
Developers of User and Carer
Involvement in Education
(DUCIE) network, 156, 167
development, 77
digital storytelling, 56
disability benefits
corrective mechanisms aimed at
countering perverse effects of,
121–2
and other social allocations, 120–1
Disability Discrimination Act, 155
Disability Equality Duty, 155

disability-related workplace
adjustments, 102
'disabled worker' status, 121–2
disabling factors with mental illness,
21, 22
disconnectedness, 25
discovery, 25
discrimination, 166, 214
fighting through public opinion
and law, 95–6
discrimination in employment
at individual level, 114–15
at institutional level, 115–16
at small business level, 116
disempowerment
level of, 137–40
of mental health services users,
135
as risk factor, 141
DSM, third edition, 90–1
'Dual Diagnosis' programme, 178

E
early warning signs, 53
economic crisis
for people with disabilities, 100
education, 51
educational attainment, 114–15
Education for All Handicapped
Children Act, 96
e-learning initiative, 161
*EMILIA Guidebook to Supporting
Users in Learning and Vocational
Integration*, 117–18
EMILIA project, 190–3
context, 174
development after, 199
group participation in, 209–10
impact of, 205–6, 206–8
intervention, 178–9
intervention at the
Middlesex demonstration
site, 180–5
method, 116–18
obstacles and facilitators
encountered during
implementation, 119
obstacles at various sites, individual
level, 118–20

234 *Index*

EMILIA project – *continued*
organisations participating in, 117
PRET and SIRC implementation
checklists, 125–7
EMILIA providers
process of intervention by, 199
EMILIA training programmes, 179
for other deprived groups, 199–200
emotionally anorexic, 195
employee and service-user roles, 66
employment, 66, 99–100
outcomes, 114
of professionals in recovery, 67
supported, 100–2
Employment and Support Allowance
in 2008, 105
'Empowering in Recovery'
programme, 178
empowerment, 26–8, 38, 209–13
defined, 136–7
evidence base for, 141–3
level of, 137–40
policy context, 140–1
reduction, 141
of schizophrenia patients, 142
Empowerment Scale, 56
engagement, 76
environmental modifications, 87
EQOLISE, 100–1
Equivalent or Lower Degree
Qualification (ELQ) framework,
166
Estroff, S.E., 21
EU
legislation for mental illnesses,
95
European IPS project, multisite, 115.
see also individual placement and
support (IPS) programmes
European lifelong learning
policy, 189
Europe's policy context for lifelong
learning, 174–5
evidence based approach to individual
placement and Support
background, 99–100
experiential expertise, 37–8
experiential knowledge, 37–8, 40,
44, 47. *see also* TREE programme

F
'Family/Network Support' Training
programme, 178
Feinstein, L., 185
Ferlie, E., 194
fighting spirit, 180
Fineman, S., 194–5
Foster, S., 160, 163–4
*Foundation for Sheltered Housing
accommodation*, 48
France
lifelong learning in, 175–6
Frankl, V.E., 181–2

G
Gell, C., 160, 163–4
General Social Care Council, 166
global functioning, 114
Greece
lifelong learning in, 175
Griffiths, C., 173–85

H
Hammond, C., 185
Handy, C., 193–4
Health Trusts in England, 72
higher education
mental health and, 154–5
Higher Education Academy, 166
high-quality care, 152
hope, 51, 71, 137
human rights protection, 151
Hutton, P., 162

I
iatrogenic injury, 22
Implementing Recovery
Organisational Change (ImROC)
Project, 72, 78–9. *see also*
organisational changes
Inclusion Institute, 167
individual empowerment, 137.
see also empowerment
individual placement and support (IPS)
evidence for, 100–2
implementation, 103–5
implementation in Nottingham, 105–6
IPS fidelity scale, 102–3
practicing, 103

individual placement and support (IPS) programmes, 113–14
in Europe, 116
with work-related social skills training, 114
individual recovery plans, 18
Individuals with Disabilities Education Act, 96
information and resources, access to, 152–3
institutional level, 88
interactional empowerment, 137
'Interactive European Lifelong Learning Programmes,' 205
International School for Communities, Rights and Inclusion (ISCRI), 167
interpersonal relationships, 88
IPS. *see* individual placement and support (IPS)
IPS fidelity scale, 102–3
Italy
mental health reform in, 92

J
job acquisition
work history for, 115
job descriptions, 66
job search, 102
Jormfeldt, H., 142

K
Kuhn, Thomas, 18

L
Lansley, Andrew, 51
law
and discrimination, 95–6
and stigma, 95–6
leaders function as role models, 103
leadership, 193
learning about involvement, 163–4
learning organisation (LO), 192
building, 193
learning skills, important, 139
Lecomte, T., 142–3
lecturers, support from, 212
Lefroy, L., 162
Lesage, A., 142–3

lifelong learning, 24–6, 122–3
courses for mental health service, 177
Danish conception of, 176
defined, 175–6
Europe's policy context for, 174–5
and higher education, 158
and mental health, 157
and recovery as a curriculum content area, 159–60
service users and carers embodying recovery and, 160–2
lifelong learning intervention
gaps in the existing, 177–8
for mental health service users, existing, 176–7
lifelong learning programmes, future aspects
barriers in the higher education setting, 165–6
funding cuts, 166
levers and opportunities, 166–7
lifelong learning programmes in other areas, 164–5
Lisbon Summit of the European Union, 112–13, 174–5
Lord, J., 142
Lutz, W.J.
definition of service empowerment by, 142

M
macroeconomic indicators, 116
Marshall, T.
on of IPS implementation, 104
meaningful choice, 139
mental distress, 214
mental health
defined, 24
and higher education, 154–5
and lifelong learning, 157
service-user trainers, 184
Mental Health Confidence Scale, 56
Mental Health Declaration for Europe, 141
Mental Health in Higher Education project, 154–5
workshop, 165
mental health policy, 155

Mental Health Policy Implementation Guide, 51
mental health services
  implication for, 72–3
  need for resources, 104
  reform, 16
  risks associated with, 21
mental health service users in
  recovery-focused services, 63–8
  as peer providers in behavioral
    health programs, 65–6
  professional stigma in, 63–5
mental health systems
  and community, policies on
    interface between, 92–4
  policies focused on, 87–92
mental health treatments,
  rehabilitation services and, 104
Mental Health Trusts, 79
Mental Health User/Consumer/
  Survivor Movement, 86
mental illness
  encouragement by practioners,
    91–2
  negative impacts of treatment and
    social environments, 23
  shift in core beliefs, 18–20
  stigma towards, 63
Mental Wealth UK project, 167
Miller, L., 105
motivational interviewing, 115
Myers, N.L., 21, 27

N
National Coordinating Centre for
  Public Engagement in higher
  education, 158
National Health Service (NHS)
  provider organisations, 72
National Institute of Adult
  Continuing Education (NIACE),
  157
National Survivor User Network
  (NSUN), 167
Nelson, G., 142
Netherlands
  TREE programme. *see* TREE
    programme in Netherlands
  user movement in psychiatry, 36–7

*Netherlands Organization for Health
  Research and Development*, 48
network sites, 79
New Economics Foundation report,
  167
New Freedom Commission on Mental
  Health, 92
New Horizons, 69
*No Health without Mental Health:
  A Cross-Government Mental Health
  Outcomes Strategy for People of All
  Ages*, 70
Non-Governmental Organisation
  [NGO]-run education, 177
Norway, 205

O
Ochoka, J., 142
Ogunleye, J., 177
Online modules on recovery, 159
online surveys
  for effective service-user
    involvement, 150
opportunity, 71
organisational changes, 74–6, 192
  approaches to, 193–5
  baseline issues, 195–6
  external obstacles, 197
  Implementing Recovery
    Organisational Change (ImROC)
    Project, 78–9
  internal obstacles, 197
  key challenges in, 76
  major issues at the 20-month point,
    197–9
  opportunities, 196–7
  prominence of user involvement,
    196
  as reflected in the focus groups,
    documentation and observations,
    195
  resistance to change, 197
Ottawa Charter on Health Promotion,
  140

P
Parnell, D., 183
part-time work, 115
passive sense of self, 25

'payoffs' for teaching staff, 160
peer-operated alternative
    programmes, 62
peer providers, mental health service
    users as, 65–6
peer support, 212
    in mental illness, 62
Perkins, R., 105
permanency of distress, 25
personal discovery, 25
personal empowerment, 27
personally informed recovery, 23–4
Personal Medicine Coaches (PMC),
    212
personal responsibility, 51
pilot sites, 79
Pinel, Philippe, 97
' Plan-Do-Study-Act' cycle for
    organisation change, 77
Poland
    lifelong learning in, 176
*Policies and practices for mental health
    in Europe – meeting the challenges*,
    140–1
policy context
    for empowerment, 140–1
post-crisis plan, 53
'post-traumatic stress support'
    programme, 178
powerful voices, 178
prejudice, 214–15
PRET implementation checklists, 125–7
professional stigma, 68. *see also*
    stigma
    towards mental illness, 63
psychiatric disabilities and TREE
    programme, 39
psychiatric hospitals, 28
psychiatric institutions, TREE
    interventions in
    informing fellow users, 41
    kick-off meeting, 41–2
    recovery self-held group, 43–4
    recovery seminar, 44–5
    starting recovery course, 45
psychiatry
    self-help in, 36
    user-initiated projects in, 36–7
    user initiatives in, 37

psychodynamic paradigm, 88
psycho-education programmes, 25
psychological empowerment, 137
Psychosis Revisited workshops, 159
psychotherapeutic relationship, 88
public opinion
    and discrimination, 95–6
    and stigma, 95–6

Q
Quality Assurance Agency, 155
quality of life (QOL), 210
    impact of empowerment on, 142

R
Reach to Recovery, 95
reclamation of life stories, 137–8
recovery, 37
    centre for mental health project, 72
    Copeland's five key principles of, 51
    defined, 37, 70–1
    problems in implementation, 71–2
    self-held group, 43–4
    seminar, 44–5
recovery course
    starting, 45
Recovery Education Program at
    the Center for Psychiatric
    Rehabilitation, 164
recovery-focused services, 67–8
recovery-orientated organisation,
    development of
    strategy development, monitoring
        and review, 77–8
    vision and benchmarking, 76–7
recovery-oriented practices by
    professionals, 73–4
recovery-oriented practitioner, 94
recovery-oriented services, 27, 69–70
Recovery Star outcome measure, 56
'Recovery-supportive care' training
    programme, 46
recurring themes, 21
*Rehabilitation '92 Foundation in the
    Netherlands*, 48
rehabilitation services and mental
    health treatments, 104
research and teaching
    service-user involvement in, 155–7

respect, 137
Reynolds, L., 161
rights
  and responsibilities for all staff, 66
  struggle for equal, 139–40
Rinaldi, M., 105
Roth, D.
  definition of service empowerment by, 142
Rowlands, J., 136

S
Sartorius, N., 22
schizoaffective disorder F25 (ICD-10), 120–1
schizophrenia, 116
Schizophrenia and Social Care, 105
schizophrenia F20 (ICD-10), 120–1
schizophrenia patients
  empowerment of, 142
schizophrenia recovery
  consumer perspective on, 23–4
secrecy to transparency, moving from, 140
self-advocacy, 51
self-confidence, 210
self-determination, 89–90, 90
self directedness, 182
self-direction, 89–90
self-disclosed disability, 67
self discovery, 138
self-efficacy
  reduction in, 141
self-esteem, 118, 211
self-help groups, 45, 138
self initiated growth, 138
self-rated functioning, 114
self-stigma, 141. *see also* stigma
  of mental health service users, 135
Senge, P., 194
service empowerment
  defined, 142
service structures, 24
service user(s), 52, 136–7
  educators, 158–61, 160
  experience of learning, 209–13
  experience of trainers, 213
  obstacles to learning, 214–15
  perceptions of empowerment, 142.
  see also empowerment

service-user involvement, 56
  access to information and resources, 152
  diversity of, 150
  high-quality care and accountability of services, 152
  human rights protection, 151
  inclusion in decision-making, 151–2
  indicators, 150–1
  involvement at and organisational/operational level, 149
  involvement at an individual level, 149–151
  involvement at a strategic level, 148–9
  making effective, 147–8
  measuring effective, 150
  organising, 150
  in teaching and research, 155–7
Shaping Our Lives, 167
sharing expertise, ongoing opportunities to, 66–7
Sheltered work, 122
Short Course in Classroom Teaching at Middlesex University, 162–3
short-course students, 165
Simpson, A., 161
SIRC implementation checklists, 125–7
SMART (Specific, Measurable, Agreed-upon, Realistic, Time-based) goals, 77–8
Smith, A., 194
social adjustment, 114
social allocations, disability benefits and other, 120–1
Social and Emotional Aspects of Learning programme in schools (SEAL), 157
'Social Competences' programme, 178
social cooperatives, 93–4
social exclusion, 28–9
social inclusion, 28–9, 71, 113–14, 209–13
socially inclusive service environs, 29–33
'Social Network' programme,' 179
social networks
  for effective service-user involvement, 150
  strength of, 142

social roles, 88
social skills, 114, 177
social support, 180
social welfare systems in Europe, 121
Social Work Education Participation
  (SWEP 2011), 155
societal attitudes
  towards mental illnesses, 96
societal empowerment, 139
Spain
  lifelong learning in, 176
staff attitudes, 104
Star of Recovery, 26
stigma, 90–1, 139, 166, 214
  fighting through public opinion
    and law, 95–6
  internalised, 116
'Strengths Approach' training
  programme, 179
structural empowerment, 139
structural equation modelling, 142
substance abuse services, 65–6
'Suicide Intervention' programme,
  179
support, 51
Supported Education model, 113–14
Supported Employment Fidelity Scale,
  103
supported employment (SE), 100–2
supported employment (SE) model,
  113–14
symptom management, 118–19
systems of care
  change in, 16–18
  individual recovery plans, 18
  recovery and citizenship, 21

T
teaching and research
  service-user involvement in, 155–7
technology
  role in service-user involvement,
    150–1
Tee, S., 162
Tew, J., 160, 163–4
Therapeutic Management of Violence
  and Aggression, 160
  training, 161–2
therapeutic nihilism, 160
thought disorder symptoms, 114

trainor, 141–2
'Train the Trainer' programme, 54
transformation, 77
treatment planning
  subordinate role in, 90
TREE effectiveness study, 48
TREE programme in Netherlands,
  38–40
  benefits of, 39–40
  future courses and training, 47–8
  informing fellow users, 41
  kick-off meeting, 41–2
  recovery self-held group, 43–4
  recovery seminar, 44–5
  'Recovery-supportive care' training
    programme, 45–6
  starting recovery course, 45
  team of, 40–1
triggers, 53
Tremblay, J., 141–2
Trimbos Institute, 48
tutoring, 214
Tuzla
  experience of service users in, 214–15

U
UK
  lifelong learning in, 175
unemployment
  young people and, 113
University of Central Lancashire
  (UCLan), 167
U.S.
  legislation for mental illnesses, 95
U.S. Substance Abuse and Mental
  Health Services Administration,
  101
User/Consumer/Survivor movement,
  87
user-developed/run recovery
  programmes, 47
user employment
  administrative difficulties, 123
'User Research Skills' programme, 179
user staff support groups, 67
user training (and certification), 66

V
Vauth, R., 141
veterans support juniors, 40

W
Wallerstein, N., 137
wellbeing, 155, 158, 167, 180
   defined, 24
Wellbeing in Higher Education
   project, 167
wellness, 52
   toolbox, 52
Wellness Recovery Action Planning
   (WRAP)
   basis of, 51
   benefits of, 55–6
   defined, 50
   development of, 51
   evaluation, 56
   features of, 52
   impact on enabling service, 56–7
   mission statement, 50–1

and national mental health policy
   in the UK, 51
overcoming the barriers, 54–6
sections, 52–4
training, 52
train the trainer programme for
   sessional workers, 54
WHO-EC partnership project, 151
work history for job
   acquisition, 115
work placements, 52
'WRAP project support,' 52

Y
young people and unemployment, 113

Z
zero exclusion, 101–2, 104